# THE ULTIMATE BODY SHAPING BIBLE

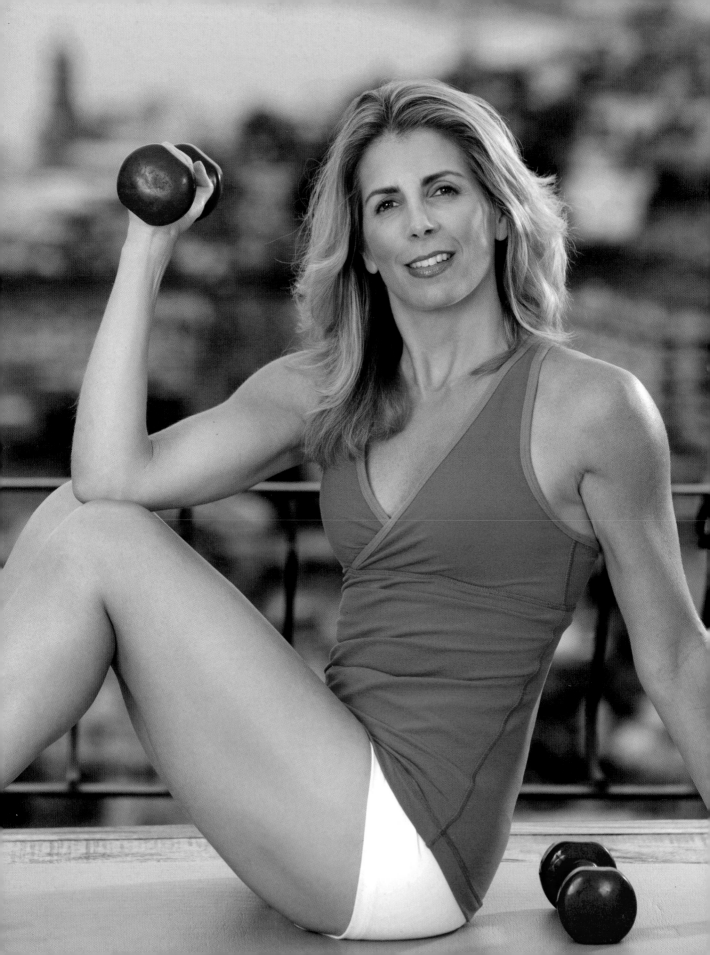

# THE

**GET IN THE BEST SHAPE OF YOUR LIFE WITH TARGETED WORKOUTS THAT TONE AND TIGHTEN EVERTHING**

# ULTIMATE BODY SHAPING BIBLE

**KARON KARTER,** author of *The Six-Week Bikini Countdown*

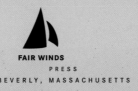

FAIR WINDS

PRESS

BEVERLY, MASSACHUSETTS

dedication
# To my mother

Text © 2009 Karon Karter

First published in the USA in 2009 by
Fair Winds Press, a member of
Quayside Publishing Group
100 Cummings Center
Suite 406-L
Beverly, MA 01915-6101
www.fairwindspress.com

13 12 11 10 09     1 2 3 4 5

ISBN-13: 978-1-59233-390-5
ISBN-10: 1-59233-390-7

Library of Congress Cataloging-in-Publication Data available


Cover and book design: Sandra Salamony
Photography: Jack Deutsch

Printed and bound in Singapore

*The information in this book is for educational purposes only. It is not intended to replace the advice of a physician or medical practitioner. Please see your health-care provider before beginning any new health program.*

# contents

# introduction

**Somewhere along the way,** muffin topping crept over your waistband while your derriere developed dimples … ouch! I get it, working off the cellulite ("eww") wasn't and isn't so simple. But I have some great news. What you did—gazillions of crunches—or didn't do—ate less bread—doesn't matter because *The Ultimate Body Shaping Bible* tones everything, yes, *everything*, from a bulging belly to back fat, droopy derriere to dumpy thighs, flabby arms to flappage anywhere on your body. This is your get-gorgeous body guide, and you'll get magnificent muscle just in time for a summer sexy body!

Why *The Ultimate Body Shaping Bible*? Because every woman has a show-it-off shape—and getting it is not as hard as you may think! You've got a hot body in there somewhere; you just need a comprehensive body plan to supertone and target your different muscle groups. With *The Ultimate Body Shaping Bible*, you'll sculpt sexy curves by combining some of the best toning exercises and calorie-scorching cardio workouts to burn the flab. Of course, a healthy diet (with normal serving sizes) is also part of the fix. Put another way: no shortcuts, no skinny-bitch tips, and no gimmicky promises—just a targeted body plan that sculpts you foxy!

Okay, you can't really spot-burn fat (hello, cardio), but you can spot-tone the areas of your body that need a little sculpting. While cardio sheds the fat, the toning exercises build strength so you can burn calories long after you've kicked off your sneakers.

## TWENTY MINUTES OF TIMELESS TERRIFIC TONERS

Muscles are the key to living dimple-free. Why? First, because muscle creates a firm base that makes fat lie flat, and second, it boosts your metabolism. With more muscle, you could possibly burn up to 45 to 50 calories a day while you're not in motion, whereas fat sits there not doing much (yeesh). Translation: burn fat every day!

Here's how it works: The workouts in this book range from beginner to super advanced, featuring a whole collection of timeless terrific toners. Each workout is about 20 minutes in length, depending on how fast you work, and each targets a specific sexy curve. Why 20 minutes? Because it's the minimum time you need to stimulate and eventually fatigue the targeted muscle you want to tone up. Within those 20 minutes, you'll do three exercises that target, for example, your outer thighs. You'll do the prescribed reps and then repeat those same exercises twice for three sets. Even though the workouts take only about 20 minutes, you should feel it, making sure you work a specific set of muscles to the point of fatigue (feel the burn) to change for the oh-so-slender better. Keep in mind

# Muscles are the key

that muscles grow when pushed to the absolute max even for a few seconds.

If, though, as you're doing the workouts, you need to rest, take one. But then keep going as long as you can to maintain good form. If you can't maintain good form, then do fewer reps. After a couple of weeks, you might not feel the work as much, and that's your clue to advance to the next workout level, because muscle grows with progressively harder work. You'll use heavier weights, resistance bands, a stability ball, and additional reps, depending on the workout. So pick your workout and workout level, do your cardio to burn excess fat first, and then do your workout. Also, do these workouts every other day so your muscles have a chance to rebuild to get your *très magnifique* body.

## SKINNY STARTS IN THE KITCHEN

Don't forget to glance at the eating tips that I provide. This is not a diet book, but a book that can help you lose about a pound a week if you just slightly alter your serving sizes and slowly switch to healthy foods. Rest assured, I don't diet and wouldn't put you through the misery. But calories count, and because skinny really starts in the kitchen, you're going to adjust what and, more specifically, how much you eat. Chances are your serving sizes are way too big, and you won't miss shaving a little off your meal as you see those jaw-dropping results!

All heart-pumping cardio sessions and eating tips are in front of each section, and the workouts are broken down into specific body areas.

To do these workouts, you'll need some inexpensive equipment—an anti-burst stability ball, about 45 to 55 centimeters wide unless you're super tall; a pair of 5-pound (2.5 kg) ankle weights, resistance bands (light, medium, and heavy), a pair of 3-pound (1.5 kg) balls, and various dumbbells. You can do these exercises inside or outside.

And just so you know, you're not the first to try these exercises. Each week, I teach a hundred or so picky (seriously) students, and they love 'em! You, too, will love these workouts for a long time to come, especially as you get fitter and foxier.

You must commit to your body. So, here's what I suggest: pay yourself for your health. Put your money on the line and pay yourself every time you work out. Pick your price—$1, $5, $10—watch it add up and then pamper—no, splurge—on *you*! (I *love* my Jimmy Choos!) A mani and pedi. Body-hugging jeans.

If you still feel stuck, check out my website, www.KaronKarterPilates.com, and email me with your questions and concerns. I'd love to hear from you! More important, we are in this together—one workout at a time—and I want you to reach your best womanly potential because you deserve it! Happy hot body!

# to living dimple-free.

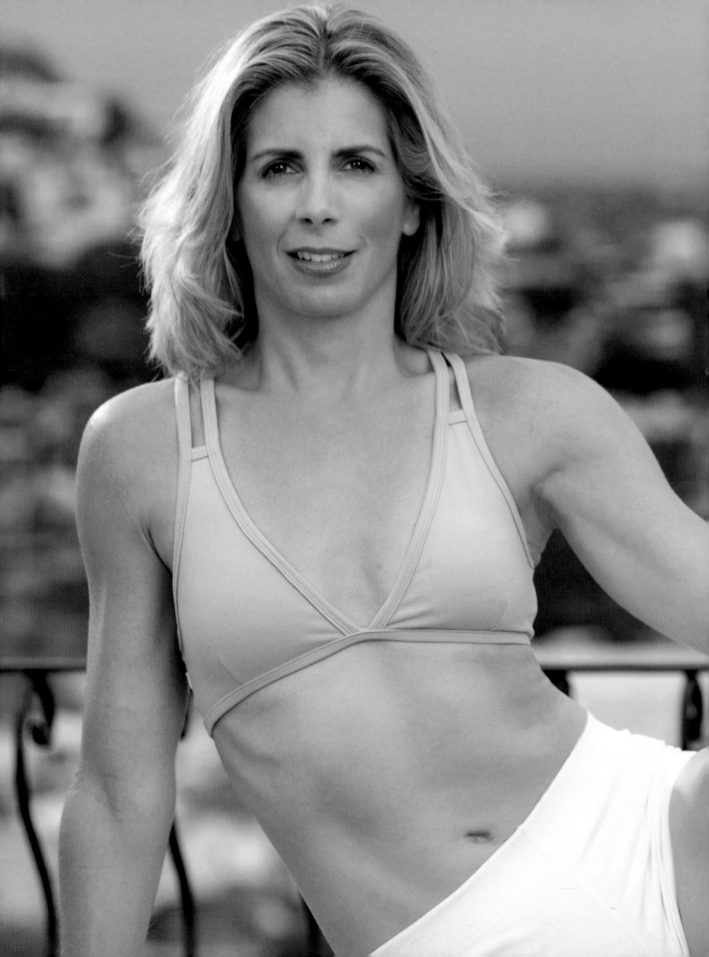

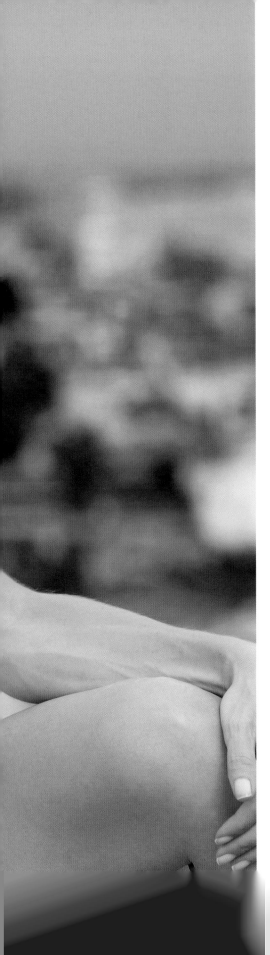

# Abs Fab-You-lous

### Cinch Your "Ultrafeminine" Waist Skinny!

**What's hot?** Let's start with what's not: muffin tops, overdone six-pack abs, paunchy or poochy *anything*. What will get you hot is a beautiful, womanly toned belly! But because the belly is notoriously stubborn in the fat department, uncovering your abs takes not a gazillion crunches but an all-out ab-attack on your midsection. This plan starts with cardio intervals to slim you down along with plenty of ab work in the following killer workouts.

Imagine turning so-so abs into *abso*-worthy— starting now, hot stuff!

# Getting to Know Your Abs

Your deepest abdominal muscle, which forms an internal girdle for your center, is called the **transversus abdominis** or transverse. Strengthening your transverse is the key to losing your belly bulge because it acts like a girdle for your lower tummy, plus it stabilizes your lumbar spine or lower back spine, keeping your back healthy.

To work your lower tummy, exhale deeply to engage your transverse—and support your lower back. As you practice and get stronger, you'll actually feel this tightening in your lower belly—or as I call it your sweet spot—from hipbone to hipbone and pubic bone to belly button. Think of zipping up your favorite pair of skinny jeans to feel your lower belly.

Next up are two sets of obliques. **Internal obliques** are deep, lying on top of your transverse, while **external obliques** are more superficial and sometimes called your six-pack muscles. Toning these muscles will provide better support for your middle, allowing you to twist and side bend at the waist, injury-free. Plus, you'll lose those love handles and back fat!

The most superficial of the group is the **rectus abdominis**, and it's a long muscle extending from your pubic bone to your sternum. When this muscle is strong, you can bend forward at the waist. All in all, your ab muscles need to be equally strong to provide support for just about any movement you do and protect your spine. Of course, your abs will look amazing, too.

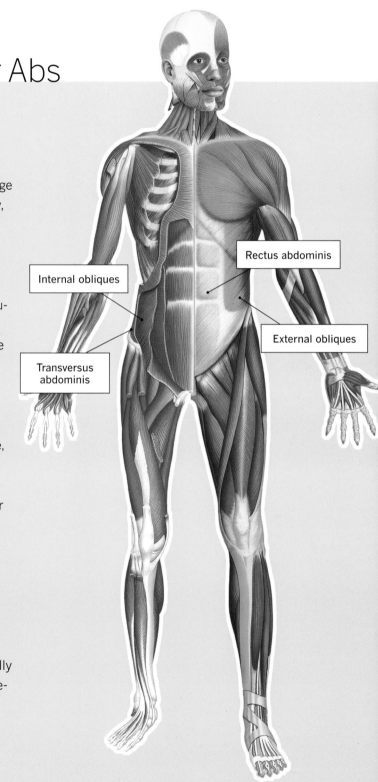

Rectus abdominis

Internal obliques

External obliques

Transversus abdominis

# Finding Neutral

Getting beautiful abs takes more than just working them out. To lose your belly bulge and protect your lower back, you'll work out with a neutral spine, i.e., good posture.

One component of a neutral spine is maintaining a neutral pelvis, so in my classes I always begin by teaching students how to hold their pelvis while doing ab moves for two reasons: first, to protect your lower back and ultimately your lumbar curve, because what happens in one part of the body will eventually affect another part; second, to work your abs to their fullest potential. Put another way, setting up your pelvis correctly means that your bones, ligaments, muscles, and discs are aligned too, which puts less stress on your spine and ensures that you won't create a belly bulge.

You'll work in a neutral pelvis in the workouts in this section. In every ab move, you must set your pelvis up correctly to build strength and protect your back, especially as you advance into the more challenging ab work. So practice moving in and out of neutral, because you're going for nothing less than amazing abs!

Finding neutral is easy with the pictures at right.

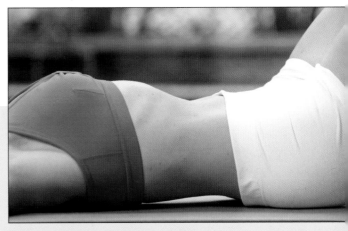

Perfect Neutral Pelvis: Your lower back is just right, and you won't create a dreaded belly bulge.

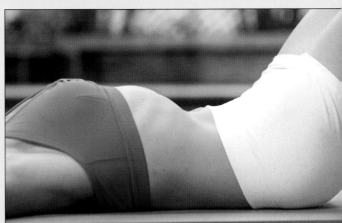

Pelvic Tilt: If your back is too flat, then your abs are slacking off and not working to their full potential.

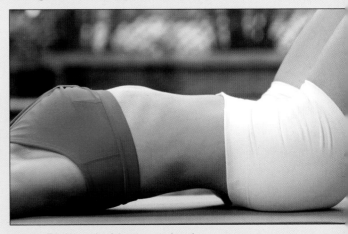

Anterior Tilt: If your back has too much arch, then you can hurt your lower back.

# Busting Your Bulge with Cardio

Burning off extra flab is the key to flat abs, and interval exercises are the best way to do it! Watch the pooch finally budge when you hit the treadmill and do one of these cardio interval sessions for 50 minutes, alternating between high-intensity (running) and low-intensity (power-walking) intervals.

To burn mega-calories, in the high-intensity intervals, your breathing should be heavy, and it should be difficult to read a magazine. In the low-intensity intervals, your heart rate must stay strong. If you feel your heart rate dropping, run a little faster or go for an all-out sprint for 30 seconds in the high-intensity interval, as in the second interval workout.

This workout is designed to be done on a treadmill, exercise bike, elliptical trainer, or stair-stepper. But if you don't have a gym membership or get bored with working out inside, do this workout outside. Just follow the times and alternate your walks and runs, or try it on a bike. Do this cardio workout four times a week.

## Cardio Workout

This workout should take 50 minutes.

**INTERVAL ONE:**
**2 minutes:** Warm up by walking 3.5 mph, no grade
**6 minutes:** Walk 4 mph, no grade
**2 minutes:** Run 5 to 6 mph, no grade

**INTERVAL TWO:**
**8 minutes:** Walk 4 mph, no grade
**2 minutes:** Run 5 to 6 mph, no grade

**INTERVAL THREE:**
**8 minutes:** Walk 4 mph, no grade
**2 minutes:** Run 5 to 6 mph, no grade

**INTERVAL FOUR:**
**8 minutes:** Walk 4 mph, no grade
**2 minutes:** Run 5 to 6 mph, no grade

**INTERVAL FIVE:**
**5 minutes:** Walk 4 mph, no grade
**2 minutes:** Run 5 to 6 mph, no grade
**2–3 minutes:** Cool down by walking 3.5 mph, no grade

# Fat Burner

If you need more of a challenge, try this fat burner.

**INTERVAL ONE:**
**2 minutes:** Warm up by walking 3.5 mph, no grade
**6 minutes:** Walk 4 mph, no grade
**2 minutes:** Run really fast (6 to 6.5 mph) so you're out of breath for about 30 seconds, and then slow down and finish with a run for 1.5 minutes, 5 to 6 mph, no grade

**INTERVAL TWO:**
**8 minutes:** Walk 4 mph, no grade
**2 minutes:** Run really fast (6 to 6.5 mph) so you're out of breath for about 30 seconds, and then slow down and finish with a run for 1.5 minutes, 5 to 6 mph, no grade

**INTERVAL THREE:**
**8 minutes:** Walk 4 mph, no grade
**2 minutes:** Run really fast (6 to 6.5 mph) so you're out of breath for about 30 seconds, and then slow down and finish with a run for 1.5 minutes, 5 to 6 mph, no grade

**INTERVAL FOUR:**
**8 minutes:** Walk 4 mph, no grade
**2 minutes:** Run really fast (6 to 6.5 mph) so you're out of breath for about 30 seconds, and then slow down and finish with a run for 1.5 minutes, 5 to 6 mph, no grade

**INTERVAL FIVE:**
**5 minutes:** Walk 4 mph, no grade
**2 minutes:** Run really fast (6 to 6.5 mph) so you're out of breath for about 30 seconds, and then slow down and finish with a run for 1.5 minutes, 5 to 6 mph, no grade
**2–3 minutes:** Cool down by walking 3.5 mph, no grade

# your belly buffet

- **BEST BELLY PORTIONS:** Slash your serving size—everything that touches your lips—by just a quarter less. Your belly won't miss it, I promise. According to *IDEA Fitness Journal,* here's what a serving size looks like: 1 cup (180 g) of cereal is about the size of your fist; one pancake is the size of a compact disc; ½ cup (75 g) fresh fruit is the size of half a baseball; 1 teaspoon (5 g) of butter is one half of a pair of dice; 1 cup (30 g) of salad greens is the size of a baseball; and 3 ounces (90 g) of meat, fish, or chicken is—get this—a deck of cards. Think you've got some shaving to do?

- **BEST BELLY FOODS:** Grapefruit, watermelon, asparagus, celery, and cucumber are all foods that make you look less puffy. Call 'em anti-bloat foods.

- **HEALTHIEST BELLY FOODS:** Spinach and dark leafy greens, which have lots of vitamin A to keep your skin looking gorgeous; salmon, which is loaded with omega-3 fatty acids, or good fats, to keep your heart healthy; lean proteins such as turkey keep you strong; avocados, packed with B vitamins that are great stress fighters; good, low-fat calcium sources such as yogurt keep your bones strong; and foods high in vitamin C, such as oranges, grapefruit, and lemons, keep you healthy and hopefully sick-free. In other words, a healthy body is a healthy belly!

- **BEST BELLY INDULGENCE:** Red wine lovers rejoice! Turns out red wine fights belly flab better than, let's say, a Cosmopolitan. I, too, occasionally enjoy a Cosmopolitan, but I used to think vodka was the only true skinny bev!

- **WORST BELLY DRINKS:** Diet colas or drinks with artificial sweeteners trick your body into wanting more calories—and bloat your belly, too (yeesh). Better belly options are water and teas of any kind (red, white, green, or black)—plus you get plenty of precious brain protectors, known as antioxidants.

# Getting a Wickedly Flat Tummy

Okay, so you're going to work off the fat with cardio four times a week and do the following lower belly exercises three times a week. Yikes! Sounds like tons of work, but keep in mind that each workout only takes about 20 minutes, so you can do these ab moves right after your cardio session. Hang in there, a beautifully toned belly is sooo worth it!

These workouts focus on all of your ab muscles—lower, middle, and upper—and your waist muscles, or internal and external obliques. Keep in mind that these workouts increase in intensity to keep your middle challenged for a long time, so focus on your form and work at your own level so as not to injure your lower back. Also, follow these important tips:

★ **Be careful.** If you have a spinal disc or lower back injury, please consult your doctor before doing any twist.

★ **Find neutral pelvis.** Don't move an inch without setting up each exercise first.

★ **Grow tall.** Lengthen your spine or think of lifting up through your pelvic floor and then twist from your bottom rib on your rib cage.

★ **Keep your head in line with your spine.** As you twist, make sure your head follows the alignment of your spine.

★ **Move from your waist.** Place your hands on your rib cage and then twist from the bottom rib. *Your hips never move; nothing moves below the waist.*

★ **Keep your back flat on the mat.** When your legs are at a 90-angle or lower, your back will be flat on the mat at all times.

★ **Focus on your sweet spot.** You should feel a tightening, similar to zipping up a pair of very tight skinny jeans, from hipbone to hipbone and pubic bone to navel.

★ **Exhale deeply.** Focus on your exhalation because it helps you strengthen your abs and protect your lower back.

★ **Do Kegels.** Your oh-so-lower tummy muscles attach from your pubic bone to your tailbone like a hammock, also known as your pelvic floor. To protect your back and beat the belly bulge, fire 'em up by pretending like you've got to go to the bathroom and there's not a restroom in sight. In other words, squeeze and hold!

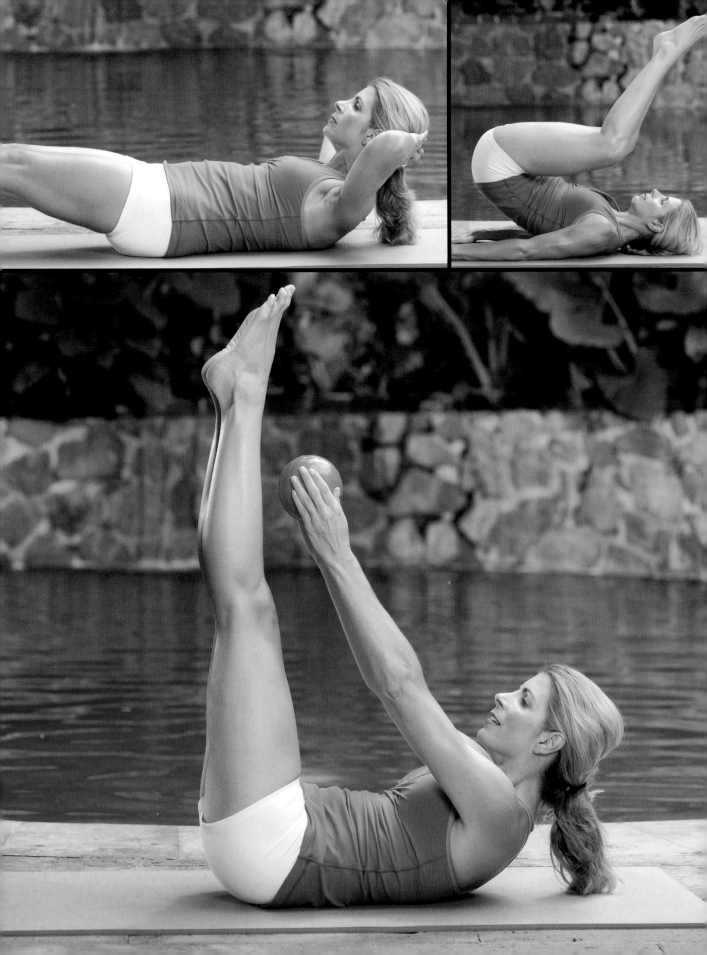

# chapter 1

# A WICKED-FLAT TUMMY

| | | the payoff | total time | how often | sets -n- reps | must-haves |
|---|---|---|---|---|---|---|
| **WORKOUT 1:**<br>beginner<br><br>Dip Your Toes<br>Reverse Curl<br>Ab-Bicycle | ○○○○ | Flattens your pooch, giving you tummy-tuck results! | 15 to 20 minutes | Do this workout 3 times a week on non-consecutive days, such as Mon., Wed., and Fri. | Do three sets of 5 to 8 reps. | Nothing |
| **WORKOUT 2:**<br>intermediate<br><br>Ab-Froggy<br>Ab-Heel Pushes<br>Straight-Leg Scissors | ○○○○ | Busts your belly bulge! | 15 to 20 minutes | Do this workout 3 times a week on non-consecutive days, such as Mon., Wed., and Fri. | Do three sets of 8 to 10 reps. | Nothing |
| **WORKOUT 3:**<br>advanced<br><br>Double Straight-Leg Lifts<br>Big Heel Beats<br>Reach and Curl with 3-pound<br>  (1.5-kg) Ball | ○○○○ | Takes you from so-so abs to fabulously flat! | 15 to 20 minutes | Do this workout 3 times a week on non-consecutive days, such as Mon., Wed., and Fri. | Do three sets of 10 to 12 reps. | 3-pound (1.5 kg) ball |
| **WORKOUT 4:**<br>super advanced<br><br>Double Straight-Leg Lifts<br>  with 3-pound (1.5-kg) Ball<br>Ferris Wheel<br>Helicopter | ○○○○ | Delivers smoking flat bikini-ready abs! | 15 to 20 minutes | Do this workout 3 times a week on non-consecutive days, such as Mon., Wed., and Fri. | Do three sets of 10 to 12 reps. | 3-pound (1.5 kg) ball |

## WORKOUT 1:
# beginner

dip your toes
reverse curl
ab-bicycle

**THE PAYOFF:**
## Flattens your pooch, giving you tummy-tuck results!

**TOTAL TIME:** 15 to 20 minutes

**HOW OFTEN:** Spend 2 to 4 weeks strengthening your transverse (lower tummy muscles) and learn how to work in a neutral pelvis to protect your lower back. Do this workout three times a week on nonconsecutive days.

★ **GETTING A WICKEDLY FLAT TUMMY,**
on page 15, offers more advice
for maximizing this workout.

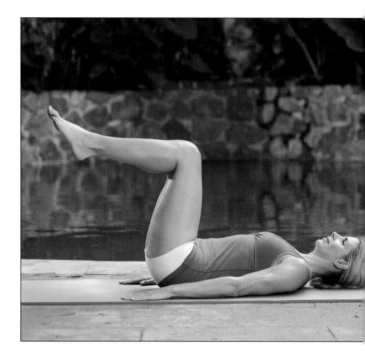

**STARTING POSITION:** Lie on your back with your knees bent at a 90-degree angle or directly in line with your hipbones. Flatten your lower back on the mat by engaging your lower tummy muscles. Straighten your arms by your sides, lengthening your fingertips. Drop the back of your shoulders against the mat, and slide your shoulders away from your ears. As you exhale, feel the tightening in your lower tummy.

## the payoff:
Tones and tightens your
lower belly

**sets -n- reps:** Do three sets of 5 to 8 reps.
**must-haves:** Nothing

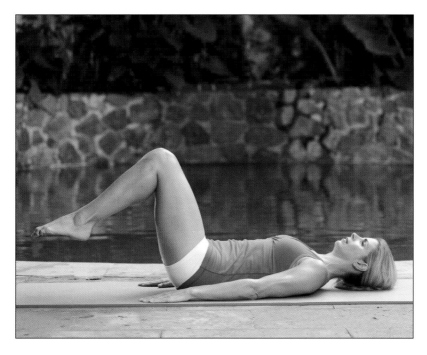

**POSITION 1:** Inhale to lower all ten toes to the floor.

**POSITION 2:** Exhale and bring your knees to the starting position. Stabilize your pelvis as your legs move. Do 5 to 8 reps.

## FABULOUS FORM TIPS

❍ Don't let your lower back come off the mat as your legs move away from your tummy. Engage your abs to melt your spine to the mat.

❍ Focus on your sweet spot.

❍ Exhale as you bring your knees into your body (starting position); otherwise, you'll miss out on tons of lower tummy work.

❍ Maintain your neutral pelvis to create a flat tummy. Working with good form strengthens your lower belly, and it also flattens your pooch. So focus, focus, and focus on good belly alignment.

❍ If you feel any tension in your lower back or can't flatten your lower back to the mat, try moving your right leg only and then your left leg for single-leg toe dips.

# **1** reverse curl

**sets -n- reps:** Do three sets of 5 to 8 reps.
**must-haves:** Nothing

○○○○

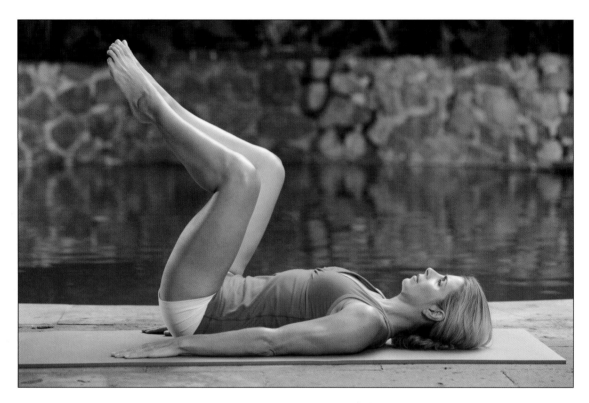

**STARTING POSITION:** Lie on your back with your knees in the air, bent and open to the side, about shoulder-width apart. Straighten your arms by your sides, lengthening your fingertips. Drop the back of your shoulders against the mat, and slide your shoulders away from your ears.

## the payoff:
Gives you tummy-tuck results!

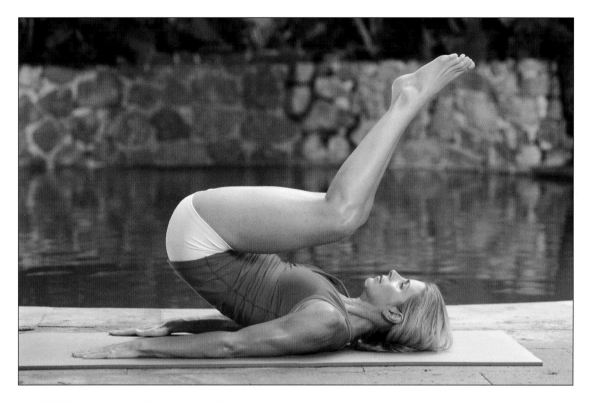

**POSITION 1:** Inhale to lift your hips off the mat.

**POSITION 2:** In the same movement, exhale to lower your hips to the mat, feeling your lower belly. Do 5 to 8 reps.

## FABULOUS FORM TIPS

○ Don't do this exercise if you have a neck or upper back injury. In addition, if you have high blood pressure or a condition called macular degeneration, check with your doctor. Any pressure on your head, neck, and shoulders may not be appropriate for you.

○ Don't drop your butt; exhale deeply to feel your lower belly work, pressing the back of your arms into the mat and reaching your fingertips long to lower your hips with control.

○ Don't lift or turn your head as you roll down; engage your abs to give you extra power.

# **1** ab-bicycle

○○○○

| | |
|---|---|
| **sets -n- reps:** | Do three sets of 5 to 8 reps. |
| **must-haves:** | Nothing |

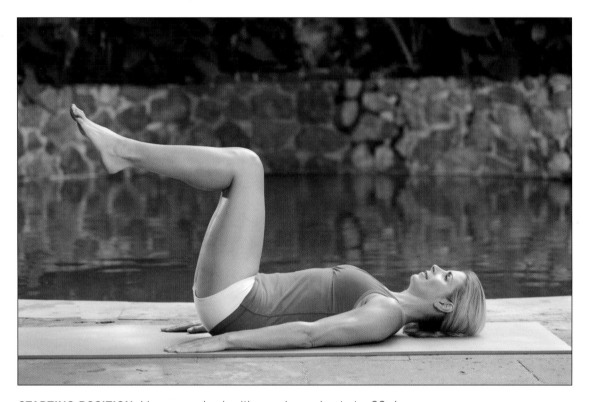

**STARTING POSITION:** Lie on your back with your knees bent at a 90-degree angle or directly in line with your hipbones. Flatten your lower back on the mat by engaging your lower tummy muscles. Straighten your arms by your sides, lengthening your fingertips. Drop the back of your shoulders against the mat, and slide your shoulders away from your ears.

## **the payoff:**

Battles your belly bump!

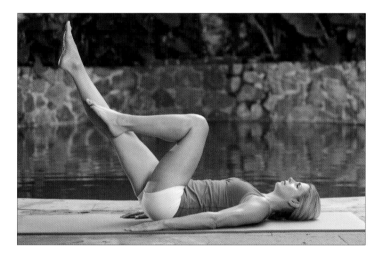

**POSITION 1:** Inhale to straighten your right leg so your toes are in line with your nose.

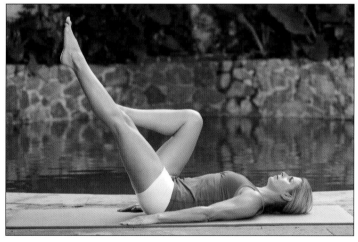

**POSITION 2:** Exhale to straighten your left leg so your toes are in line with your nose. Continuously move your legs for 8 reps and then switch your breath work so you begin with the left leg—inhale and then exhale on the right leg for 8 reps.

## FABULOUS FORM TIPS

❍ Don't let your lower back come off the mat as you cycle your legs.

❍ Don't move your pelvis; use your lower belly muscles to stabilize your pelvis as your legs move continuously to challenge your lower tummy muscles. Exhales help stabilize, so use 'em.

❍ Lower your legs if you need more tummy work. If, however, you feel strain in your lower back, raise your legs higher. Toes to the ceiling makes the work easier for your belly and back.

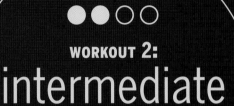

**WORKOUT 2:**
# intermediate

ab-froggy
ab-heel pushes
straight-leg scissors

**THE PAYOFF:**
## Busts your belly bulge !

**TOTAL TIME:** 15 to 20 minutes

**HOW OFTEN:** Spend two to four weeks focusing on feeling your sweet spot so you can literally feel your lower tummy working, plus you're still strengthening your transverse. Do this workout three times a week on nonconsecutive days.

★ **GETTING A WICKEDLY FLAT TUMMY,** on page 15, offers more advice for maximizing this workout.

# **2** ab-froggy

○○○○

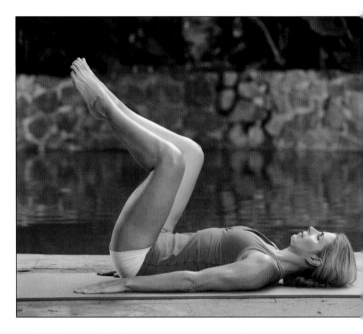

**STARTING POSITION:** Lie on your back with your knees in the air, bent and open to the side, about shoulder-width apart. Glue your heels together and flex your feet. Your lower back should be flat on the floor, engaging your lower tummy muscles. Straighten your arms by your sides, lengthening your fingertips. Drop the back of your shoulders against the mat, and slide your shoulders away from your ears.

## the payoff:
Busts your belly bulge!

**sets -n- reps:** Do three sets of 8 to 10 reps.
**must-haves:** Nothing

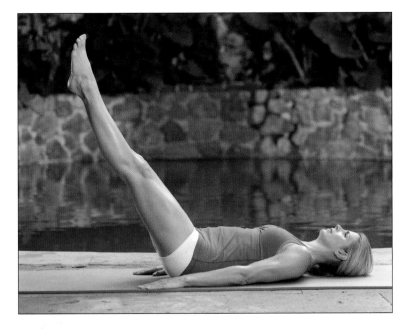

**POSITION 1:** Inhale to straighten your legs so your toes are in line with your nose.

**POSITION 2:** Exhale and return your knees to the starting position. Stabilize your pelvis as your legs move. Do 8 to 10 reps.

## FABULOUS FORM TIPS

○ Don't let your lower back come off the mat, especially as your legs move away from your middle, challenging your belly muscles.

○ Don't forget to exhale as you bring your legs into your body. You want to feel your sweet spot!

○ Squeeze your inner thighs as you straighten your legs to sneak in some inner thigh toning; if you can't straighten your legs, do what you can but never move your pelvis. After all, you don't want to create a belly bulge.

# 2 ab-heel pushes

**sets -n- reps:** Do three sets of 8 to 10 reps.
**must-haves:** Nothing

○○○○

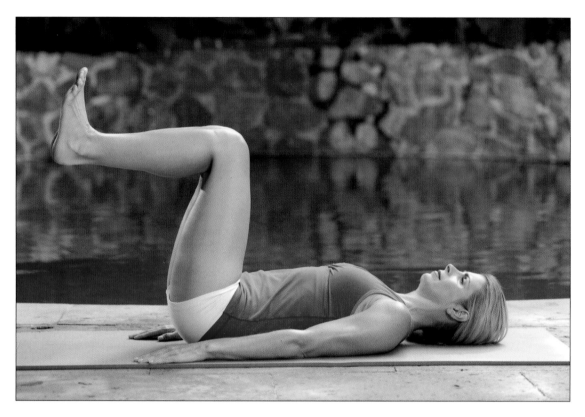

**STARTING POSITION:** Lie on your back with your knees bent at a 90-degree angle, knees touching, and feet parallel and flexed. Flatten your lower back on the mat, engaging your lower tummy muscles. Straighten your arms by your sides, lengthening your fingertips. Drop the back of your shoulders against the mat, and slide your shoulders away from your ears.

## the payoff:

Uncovers "La Bella" belly!

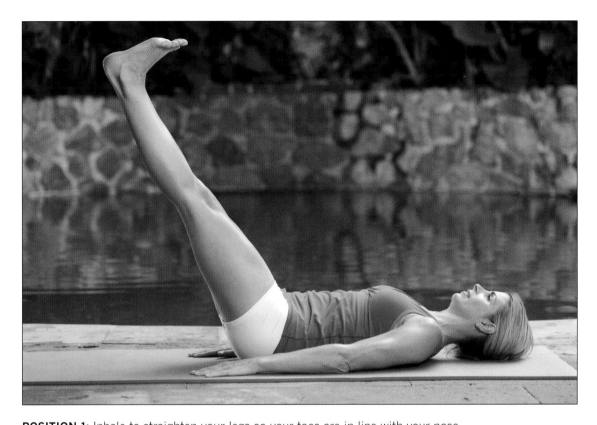

**POSITION 1:** Inhale to straighten your legs so your toes are in line with your nose.

**POSITION 2:** Exhale and return your knees to the starting position. Imagine you're pushing against a wall to engage your abs completely. Don't move your pelvis while your legs move. Do 8 to 10 reps.

## FABULOUS FORM TIPS

○ Don't let your lower back come off the mat, especially as your legs move away from your body, challenging your belly muscles.

○ Don't forget to exhale as you bring your legs into your body. You want to feel your sweet spot!

○ Squeeze your inner thighs as you straighten your legs to sneak in some inner thigh toning; if you can't straighten your legs, do what you can but never move your pelvis. After all, you don't want to create a belly bulge.

# 2 straight-leg scissors

○○○○

**sets -n- reps:** Do three sets of 8 to 10 reps.
**must-haves:** Nothing

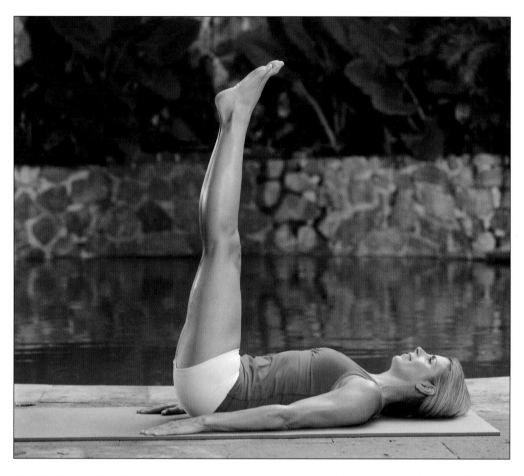

**STARTING POSITION:** Lie on your back with your legs straight lengthening to the ceiling at a 90-degree angle or in line with your hipbones. Flatten your lower back on the mat, engaging your lower tummy muscles. Straighten your arms by your sides, lengthening your fingertips. Drop the back of your shoulders against the mat, and slide your shoulders away from your ears.

## the payoff:

Tones your tummy like really fast!

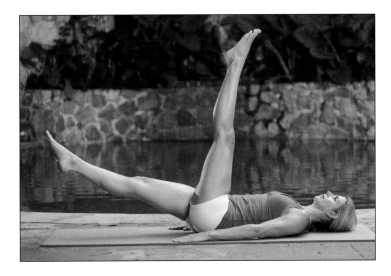

**POSITION 1:** Inhale to drop your right leg to the floor so your toes are in line with your nose, but don't lower your foot to the floor. Make your tummy work.

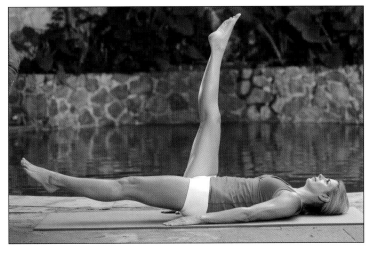

**POSITION 2:** Exhale to switch legs scissor-like so your right leg lifts to the ceiling and your left to the floor, but don't touch it if you want to engage your lower tummy. Imagine scissoring your legs as if a piece of glass is between your legs. Do 8 to 10 reps.

## FABULOUS FORM TIPS

○ Don't bounce your torso as you scissor your legs; establish a continuous smooth tempo with each exhale.

○ Don't bend your knees; keep your legs straight if you can. Sometimes, tight hamstrings prevent you from straightening your legs. Eventually, you'll get there!

# WORKOUT 3:
## advanced

●●●○

double straight-leg lifts
big heel beats
reach and curl with
3-pound (1.5 kg) ball

**THE PAYOFF:**
## Takes you from so-so abs to fabulously flat!

**TOTAL TIME:** 15 to 20 minutes

**HOW OFTEN:** Spend two to four weeks
strengthening your lower tummy muscles.
Do this workout three times a week
on nonconsecutive days.

★ **GETTING A WICKEDLY FLAT TUMMY,**
on page 15, offers more advice
for maximizing this workout.

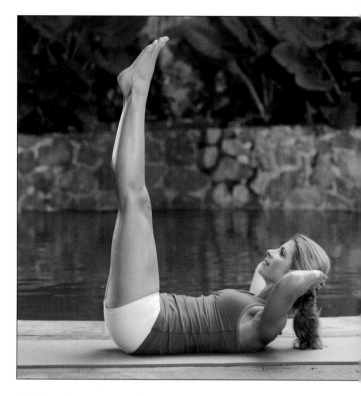

**STARTING POSITION:** Lie on your back with straight
legs lengthening to the ceiling at a 90-degree angle
or in line with your hipbones. Clasp your hands and
place them behind your head. Lift your shoulders off
the ground, and curl your chin to your chest. Flatten
your lower back on the mat, engaging your lower
tummy muscles.

## the payoff:
Gives you a flat-tastic
tummy!

# leg lifts

**sets -n- reps:** Do three sets of 10 to 12 reps.
**must-haves:** Nothing

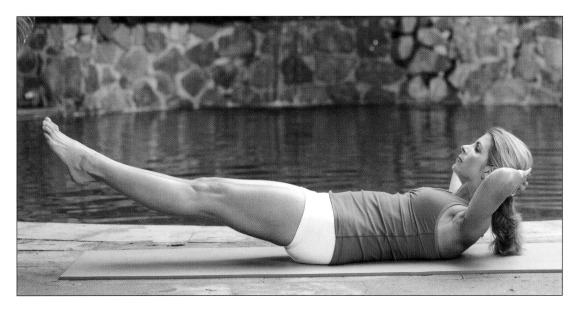

**POSITION 1:** Inhale to lower your legs to the floor, only taking your legs as low as your lower back stays anchored to the mat: no strain, no arch, no bulge! Don't lift your lower back off the mat; lower your legs as low as your back allows.

**POSITION 2:** Exhale to lift your legs back to the 90-degree angle, exhaling out every last breath to drop your belly button to your spine. Do 10 to 12 reps.

## FABULOUS FORM TIPS

○ Engage your sweet spot! At this advanced level, you should feel the tightening around your lower belly every time.

○ Exhale to protect your lower back and seriously strengthen your lower tummy.

○ Imagine a lap belt tightly fastened around your lower belly, from hipbone to hipbone, to feel your lower belly muscles or transverse.

# **3** big heel beats

**sets -n- reps:** Do three sets of 10 to 12 reps.
**must-haves:** Nothing

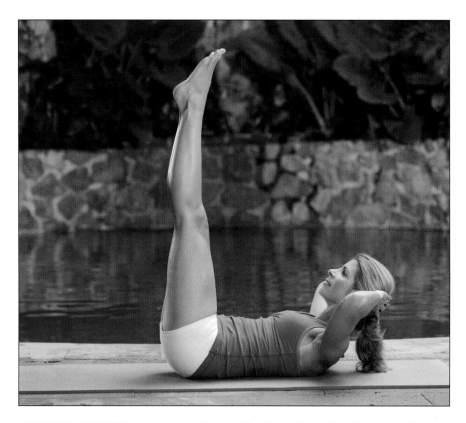

**STARTING POSITION:** Lie on your back with straight legs lengthening to the ceiling at a 90-degree angle or in line with your hipbones. Clasp your hands and place them behind your head. Lift your shoulders off the ground, and curl your chin to your chest.

## **the payoff:**

Bulge begone!

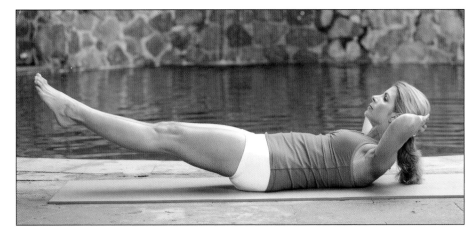

**POSITION 1:** Inhale to lower your legs to the floor, taking your legs as low as your lower back stays anchored to the mat: no strain, no arch, no bulge! Don't lift your lower back off the mat; lower your legs as low as your back allows.

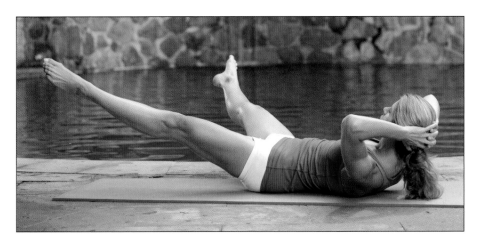

**POSITION 2:** Inhale to open your legs, about shoulder-width apart, and then exhale to close your legs, exhaling out every last breath to drop your belly button to your spine. Do 10 to 12 reps.

## FABULOUS FORM TIPS

❍ Contract your pelvic floor as you open and close your legs; imagine having to use the bathroom, but there's not a restroom in sight. Squeeze and hold it!

❍ Engage your sweet spot. It's a must!

# **3** reach and curl with 3-pound ball

○○○○

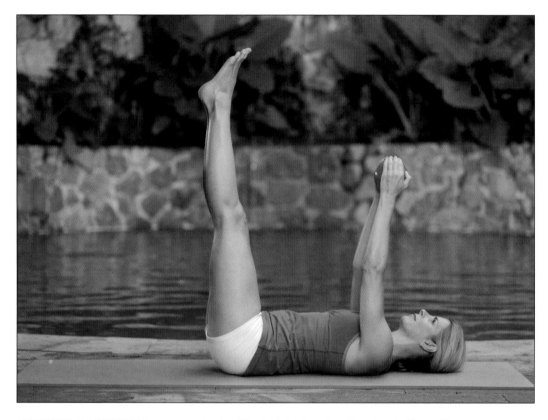

**STARTING POSITION:** Lie on your back with straight legs lengthening to the ceiling at a 90-degree angle or in line with your hipbones. With your head on the mat, hold a 3-pound (1.5-kg) ball in your hands, and straighten your arms over your nose.

## **the payoff:**

Tones your tummy—so flat—I promise!

**sets -n- reps:** Do three sets of 10 to 12 reps.
**must-haves:** 3-pound (1.5-kg) ball

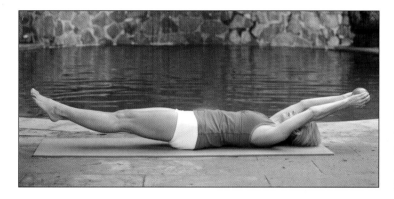

**POSITION 1:** Inhale to lower your legs to the floor while your arms are behind your head. Remember, no strain, no arch, no bulge. Don't lift your lower back off the mat; only lower your legs as low as your back allows.

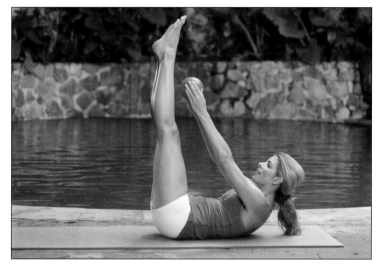

**POSITION 2:** Then exhale to lift your legs and arms so your head, neck, and shoulders come off the mat. Then lower your arms and legs to the floor. Do 10 to 12 reps.

## FABULOUS FORM TIPS

○ Engage your sweet spot! At this advanced level, you should feel the tightening around your lower belly every time.

○ Exhale to protect your lower back and seriously strengthen your lower tummy.

○ Don't strain your neck. Drop the weighted ball if you feel any neck strain.

○ Don't forget to really curl up—reaching the ball toward your toes to get yummy belly work.

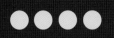

**WORKOUT 4:**

# super advanced

double straight-leg lifts
with 3-pound (1.5 kg) ball
ferris wheel
helicopter

---

**THE PAYOFF:**
## Delivers smoking flat bikini-ready abs!

---

**TOTAL TIME:** 15 to 20 minutes

**HOW OFTEN:** Honestly, you're there! Work at this level as long as you want to keep your abs shapely and strong. Do this workout three times a week on nonconsecutive days.

★ **GETTING A WICKEDLY FLAT TUMMY,**
**on page 15, offers more advice**
**for maximizing this workout.**

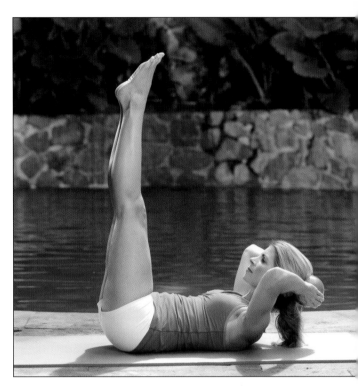

**STARTING POSITION:** Lie on your back with straight legs lengthening to the ceiling at a 90-degree angle. Clasp a 3-pound (1.5 kg) ball in your hands and place them behind your head. Lift your shoulders off the ground, and curl your chin to your chest.

## the payoff:
Shapely and strong abs!

# leg lifts with 3-pound ball

**sets -n- reps:** Do three sets of 10 to 12 reps.
**must-haves:** 3-pound (1.5-kg) ball

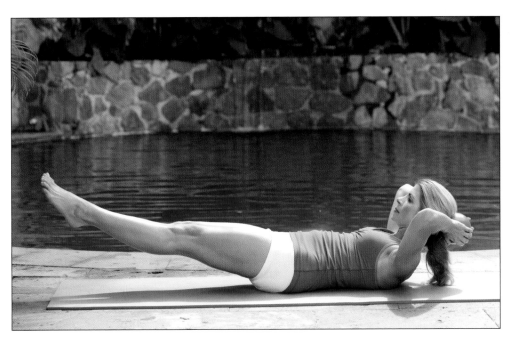

**POSITION 1:** Inhale to lower your legs to the floor, only taking the legs as low as your lower back stays anchored to the mat: no strain, no arch, no bulge! Don't lift your lower back off the mat; only lower your legs as low as your back allows.

**POSITION 2:** Exhale to lift your legs to a 90-degree angle, exhaling out every last breath to drop your belly button to your spine. Do 10 to 12 reps.

## FABULOUS FORM TIPS

❍ Engage your sweet spot! At this advanced level, you should feel the tightening around your lower belly every time.

❍ Imagine a lap belt tightly fastened around your lower belly, from hipbone to hipbone, to feel your lower belly muscles or transverse.

❍ Exhale to protect your lower back and seriously strengthen your lower tummy.

❍ Don't tense your neck. Drop the weighted ball if you feel any neck strain.

# **4** ferris wheel

○○○○

**sets -n- reps:** Do three sets of 10 to 12 reps.
**must-haves:** Nothing

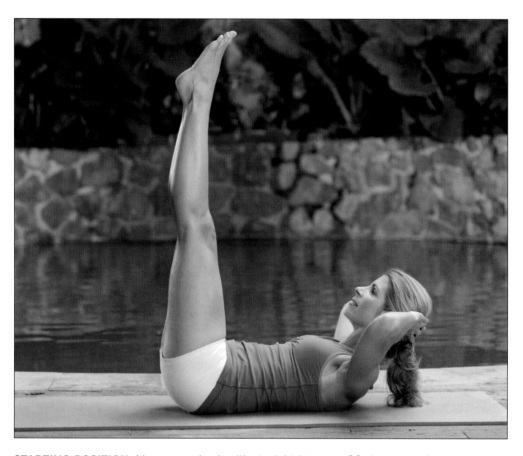

**STARTING POSITION:** Lie on your back with straight legs at a 90-degree angle.
Clasp your hands and place them behind your head. Lift your shoulders off the
ground, and curl your chin to your chest.

## the payoff:

Uncovers the sexy belly down deep!

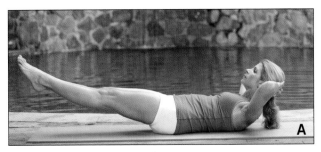

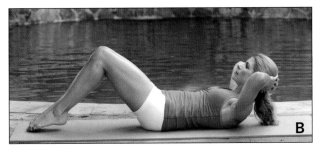

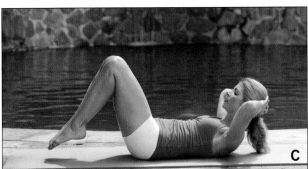

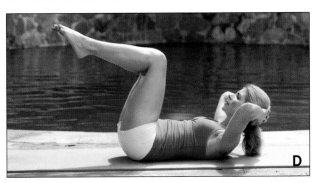

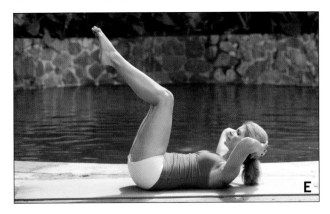

**POSITION 1:** Inhale to lower your legs to the floor. Don't lift your lower back off the mat; only lower your legs as low as your back allows. Imagine reaching your toes way away from your body (A).

**POSITION 2:** Exhale to bend your knees and drag your toes along the mat (B).

**POSITION 3:** Keep moving your legs into your body (really use your tummy) and then up to the starting position, engaging your lower tummy (C–E). Do 10 to 12 reps.

## FABULOUS FORM TIPS

❍ Engage your sweet spot! At this advanced level, you should feel the tightening around your lower belly every time.

❍ Exhale to protect your lower back and seriously strengthen your lower tummy.

# 4 helicopter

○○○○

**sets -n- reps:** Do three sets of 10 to 12 reps.
**must-haves:** Nothing

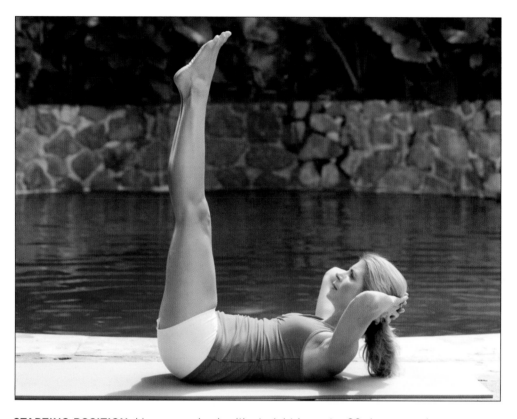

**STARTING POSITION:** Lie on your back with straight legs at a 90-degree angle. Clasp your hands and place them behind your head. Lift your shoulders off the ground, and curl your chin to your chest.

## the payoff:

Bye-bye big belly! Hello flat tummy!

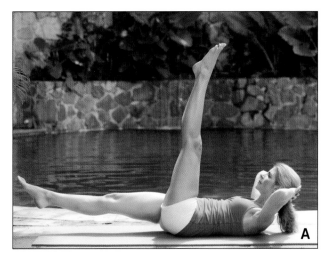

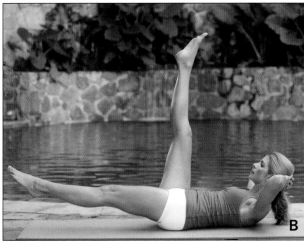

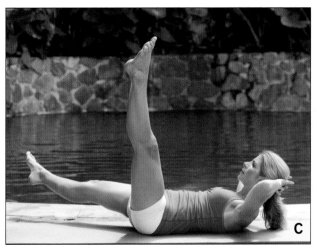

**POSITION 1:** Inhale to lower your right leg to just about 4 inches (10 cm) off the floor while your left leg lengthens to the ceiling.

**POSITION 2:** Switch your legs like a pair of scissors so your left leg is now about 4 inches (10 cm) off the floor.

**POSITION 3:** Exhale to open and circle your legs out to the sides, wider than your shoulders, keeping 'em about 4 inches (10 cm) off the floor. (Imagine a propeller of a helicopter.) Feel the lower tummy work as you circle your legs. Repeat the exercise with your left leg down and right leg up; that completes one set of helicopters. Do 10 to 12 reps.

# FABULOUS FORM TIPS

○ Don't bounce your torso as you scissor your legs; establish a smooth tempo with each movement.

○ Don't lift your lower back off the mat as you helicopter your legs.

○ Use your pelvic floor muscles. Imagine having to use the bathroom, but there's not a restroom in sight. Squeeze and hold it.

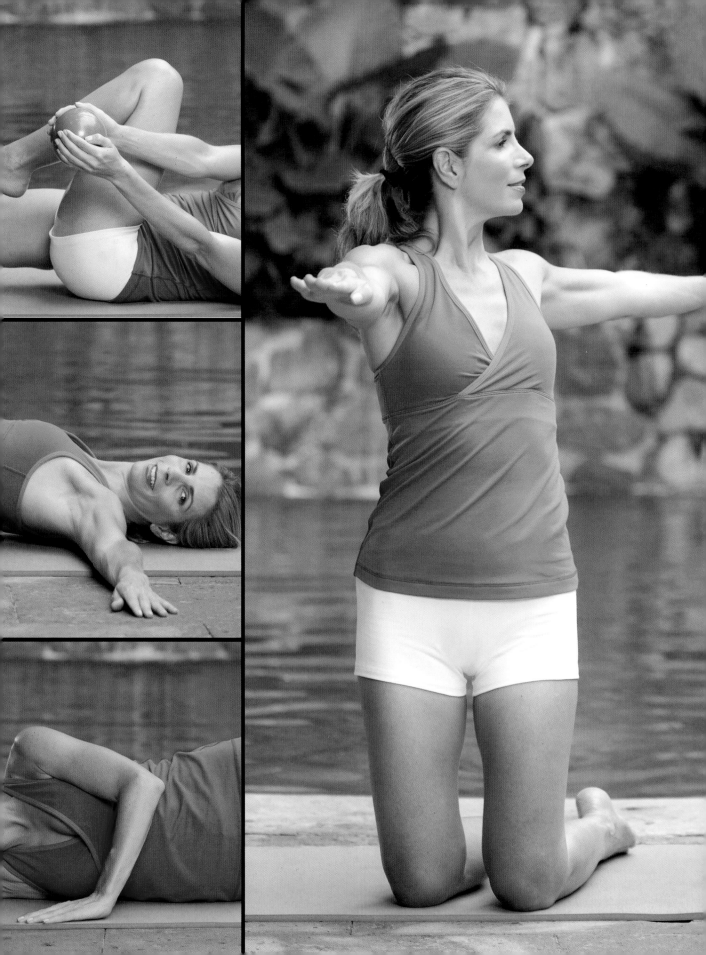

# chapter 2

# DE-WIGGLE YOUR MIDDLE

| | | the payoff | total time | how often | sets -n- reps | must-haves |
|---|---|---|---|---|---|---|
| **WORKOUT 1:**<br>beginner<br><br>Oblique Twist<br>Windshield Wiper Legs (Knees)<br>Oblique Twist on Knees | ○○○○ | Handles your love handles! | 15 to 20 minutes | Do this workout 3 times a week on non-consecutive days, such as Mon., Wed., and Fri. | Do three sets of 5 to 8 reps. | Nothing |
| **WORKOUT 2:**<br>intermediate<br><br>Can Can<br>Criss-Cross<br>Windshield Wiper (Straight) Legs | ○○○○ | Gives you an itty-bitty waist! | 15 to 20 minutes | Do this workout 3 times a week on non-consecutive days, such as Mon., Wed., and Fri. | Do three sets of 8 to 10 reps. | Not a thing, ladies! |
| **WORKOUT 3:**<br>advanced<br><br>Corkscrew<br>Reach and Twist with<br>  3-pound (1.5-kg) Ball<br>Straight Line Side Lifts | ○○○○ | Takes lotsa inches off your waist! | 15 to 20 minutes | Do this workout 3 times a week on non-consecutive days, such as Mon., Wed., and Fri. | Do three sets of 10 to 12 reps. | 3-pound (1.5-kg) ball |
| **WORKOUT 4:**<br>super advanced<br><br>Reach and Twist with Straight Legs<br>  (3-pound [1.5-kg] Ball)<br>Straight Line Side Lifts<br>  (3-pound [1.5-kg] Ball)<br>Windshield Wiper Legs (Isometric) | ○○○○ | Defines your lovely waist! | 20 minutes | Do this workout 3 times a week on non-consecutive days, such as Mon., Wed., and Fri. | Do three sets of 10 to 12 reps. | 3-pound (1.5-kg) ball |

○○○○

## WORKOUT 1:
# beginner

oblique twist
windshield wiper legs (knees)
oblique twist on knees

---

**THE PAYOFF:**
## Handles your love handles!

---

**TOTAL TIME:** 15 to 20 minutes

**HOW OFTEN:** Spend two to four weeks strengthening your waist muscles and focus on twisting correctly (using your obliques) to protect your lower back. Do this workout three times a week on nonconsecutive days.

★ **GETTING A WICKEDLY FLAT TUMMY,**
**on page 15, offers more advice**
**for maximizing this workout.**

# 1 oblique twist

○○○○

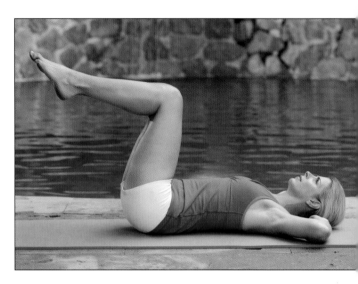

**STARTING POSITION:** Lie on your back with your knees bent at a 90-degree angle or directly in line with your hipbones. "Glue" your knees together. Clasp your hands behind your head, and slide your shoulders away from your ears.

## the payoff:
Sculpts your sides!

**sets -n- reps:** Do three sets of 5 to 8 reps.
**must-haves:** Nothing

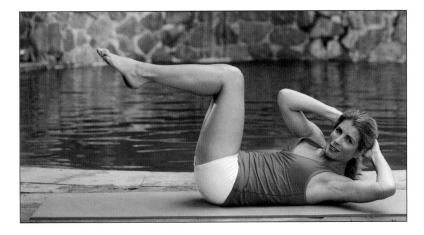

**POSITION 1:** Inhale to prepare for the movement, and then lift to twist your right elbow to your left knee. Hold this twist for three full breaths, sinking the belly deeper, twisting a little higher with each breath. Inhale to the starting position.

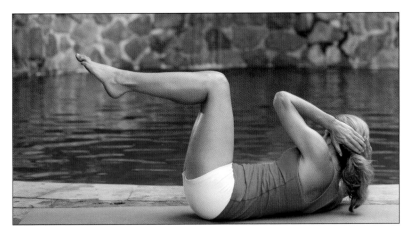

**POSITION 2:** Exhale to lift and twist your left elbow to your right knee. Do 5 to 8 reps.

## FABULOUS FORM TIPS

○ Don't move your knees. What makes this exercise so hard is the isolation of the obliques. So focus on the twist—lifting your elbow to your knee.

○ Don't move your pelvis. Your knees must remain over your hipbones to isolate the obliques.

○ Don't cheat. Move your elbow to your knee—not your knee to your elbow, because you'll miss out on the yummy waist work.

# **1** windshield wiper legs (knees)

○○○○

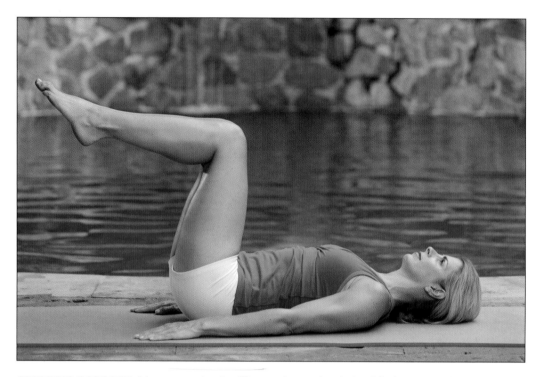

**STARTING POSITION:** Lie on your back with your knees bent at a 90-degree angle. Straighten your arms by your sides, lengthening your fingertips. Drop the back of your shoulders against the mat, and slide your shoulders away from your ears.

## **the payoff:**

Strengthens and sculpts your waist!

**sets -n- reps:** Do three sets of 5 to 8 reps.

**must-haves:** Nothing

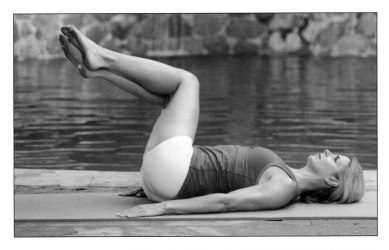

**POSITION 1:** Move your knees to the right slowly and then exhale to the starting position.

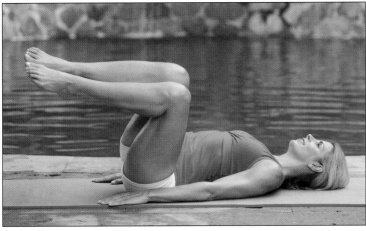

**POSITION 2:** Move your knees to the left slowly and then exhale to the starting position, focusing on the deep waist muscles. Do 5 to 8 reps.

## FABULOUS FORM TIPS

○ Don't shift your knees when you move them from side to side; keep your knees even and aligned over your hips to deepen your waist work.

○ Don't overdo the movement. Focus on your deep obliques (you may feel the work deep on the sides of your back), contracting as you move your legs from side to side.

# **1** oblique twist on knees

**sets -n- reps:** Do three sets of 5 to 8 reps.
**must-haves:** Nothing

○○○○

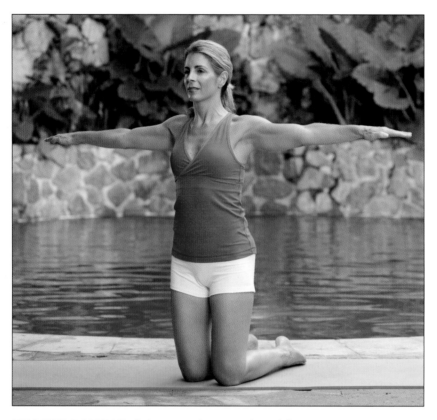

**STARTING POSITION:** Get on your knees and straighten your torso, making sure your belly button lifts to your spine. Lengthen your arms out by your sides so you're making a T shape.

## the payoff:

Defines your waist!

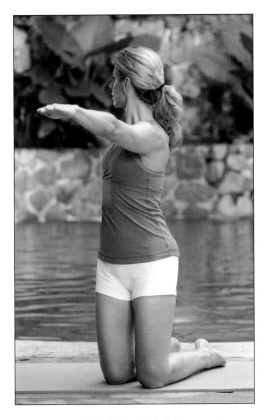 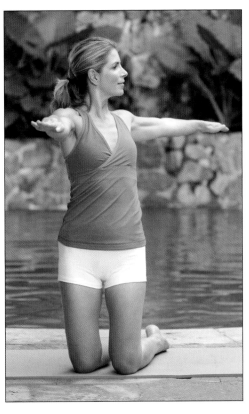

**POSITION 1:** Inhale to lift tall in your torso and then exhale to twist to the right at the waist from the last rib only.

**POSITION 2:** Inhale to the starting position and then exhale to the left side, focusing on your exhale to engage your waist muscles. Do 5 to 8 reps.

## FABULOUS FORM TIPS

❍ Don't move your hips; this twist should come from your bottom ribs to isolate your waist muscles.

❍ Work in a neutral pelvis; firm up your bottom. Imagine a pencil between your butt cheeks, but don't tuck your pelvis.

❍ Lengthen your spine; lift from your groin to grow tall in your spine before twisting.

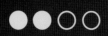

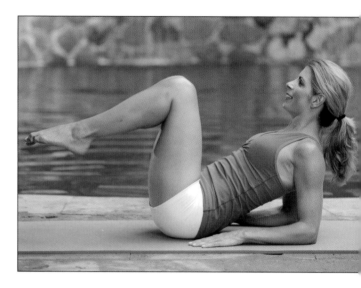

**STARTING POSITION:** Sit on your bum with your elbows bent behind you. Pull your knees to your chest and use your abs to hold them in place.

## the payoff:
Erases waist worries!

---

**WORKOUT 2:**

# intermediate

can can
criss-cross
windshield wiper
(straight) legs

---

**THE PAYOFF:**

## Gives you an itty-bitty waist!

---

**TOTAL TIME:** 15 to 20 minutes

**HOW OFTEN:** Spend two to four weeks strengthening your waist muscles so you can actually feel the contraction in your obliques; it's like your rib cage collapses around your waist. Do this workout three times a week on nonconsecutive days.

★ **GETTING A WICKEDLY FLAT TUMMY,** on page 15, offers more advice for maximizing this workout.

**sets -n- reps:** Do three sets of 8 to 10 reps.

**must-haves:** Not a thing, ladies!

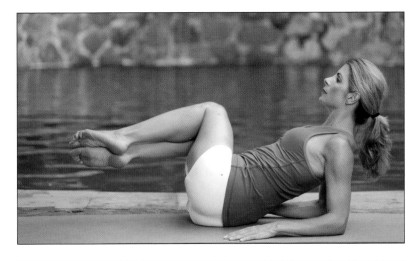

**POSITION 1:** "Glue" your knees together. Inhale to lower your knees to the right and then exhale to lift the knees to the starting position.

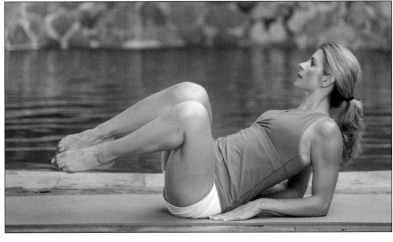

**POSITION 2:** Inhale to lower your knees to the left and then exhale to lift the knees to the starting position. Do 8 to 10 reps.

## FABULOUS FORM TIPS

○ Don't shift or move your knees; "glue" your knees together to isolate your obliques. Go for the skinny-waist work.

○ Use your exhale to move your knees to the starting position, feeling your waist muscles firing up!

○ Don't move your upper body; stabilize it and move only from your bottom ribs to super-engage the obliques.

# 2 criss-cross

○○○○

**sets -n- reps:** Do three sets of 8 to 10 reps.
**must-haves:** Not a thing, ladies!

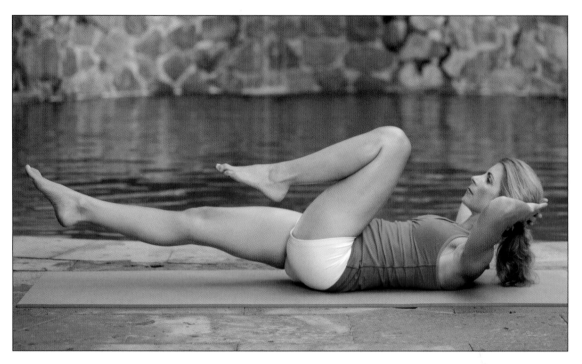

**STARTING POSITION:** Lie on your back and straighten your right leg so it's about nose level—toes in line with your nose—while your left knee is bent.

## the payoff:

Slims your waist!

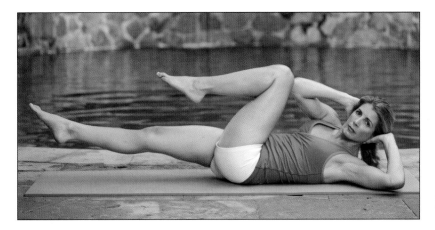

**POSITION 1:** Inhale to lift and twist your right elbow to your left knee, moving from your bottom rib.

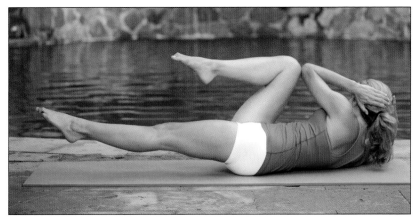

**POSITION 2:** Exhale to switch legs, lift and then twist your left elbow to your right knee, moving from your bottom rib while straightening your left leg. Do 8 to 10 reps.

# FABULOUS FORM TIPS

○ Don't move from your neck—a big no-no! Not only could you hurt the delicate neck muscles, but you're also not working your waist—so not sexy!

○ Use your tummy muscles to lift, curl, and twist.

○ Twist from your waist. Imagine wringing out your lungs with each twist.

○ Deepen your twist. Open up your elbows and reach your elbow past your knee to get the itty-bitty waist work.

# 2 windshield wiper (straight) legs

○○○○

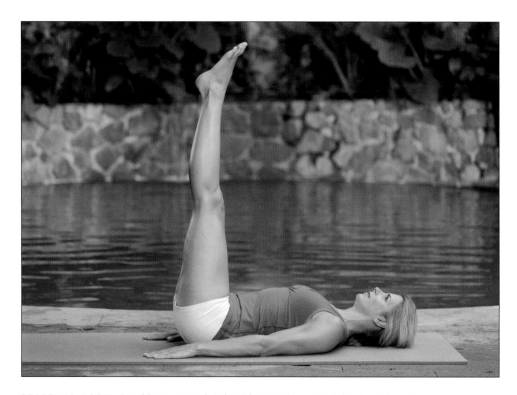

**STARTING POSITION:** Lie on your back with your legs straight, lengthening to the ceiling at a 90-angle or in line with your hipbones. Straighten your arms by your sides, lengthening your fingertips. Drop the back of your shoulders against the mat, and slide your shoulders away from your ears.

## the payoff:

Gives you lotsa-less around your middle!

**sets -n- reps:**  Do three sets of 8 to 10 reps.
**must-haves:**  Not a thing, ladies!

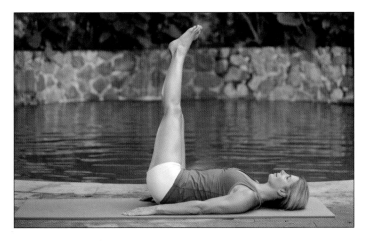

**POSITION 1:** Keeping your knees and ankles together, move your legs to the right so your hip comes off the mat slightly, and then exhale to the starting position.

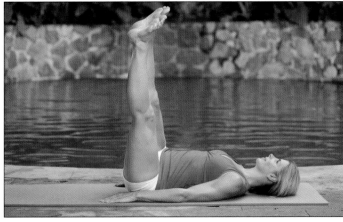

**POSITION 2:** Keeping your knees and ankles together, move your legs to the left so your hip comes off the mat slightly, and then exhale to the starting position. Do 8 to 10 reps.

## FABULOUS FORM TIPS

○ Don't lift your head or shoulders off the mat; keep the movement small until you build enough strength in the deep obliques.

○ Use your deep obliques to move your legs from side to side. Move slowly with control so you can feel this waist work.

○ Don't separate your legs. Instead, squeeze your inner thighs to give you lots of power!

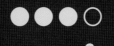

## WORKOUT 3:
# advanced

corkscrew
reach andtwist with
3-pound (1.5-kg) ball
straight line side lifts

---

### THE PAYOFF:
## Takes lotsa inches off your waist!

---

**TOTAL TIME:** 15 to 20 minutes

**HOW OFTEN:** By now, you should feel the tightening in your obliques! Spend two to four weeks to super-tone your waist. Do this workout three times a week on nonconsecutive days.

★ **GETTING A WICKEDLY FLAT TUMMY, on page 15, offers more advice for maximizing this workout.**

# 3  corkscrew
○○○○

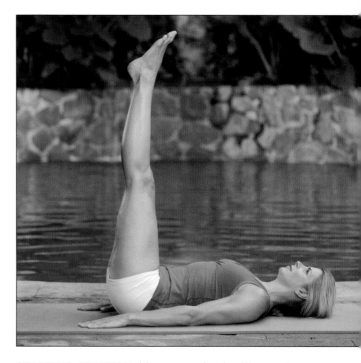

**STARTING POSITION:** Lie on your back with your legs straight, lengthening to the ceiling at a 90-degree angle or in line with your hipbones. Straighten your arms by your sides, lengthening your fingertips. Drop the back of your shoulders against the mat, and slide your shoulders away from your ears.

## the payoff:
Gives you an itty-bitty waist

**sets -n- reps:** Do three sets of 10 to 12 reps.
**must-haves:** Nothing

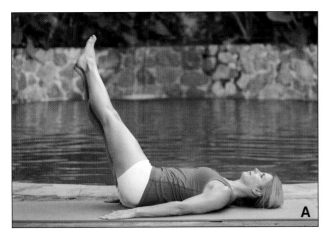

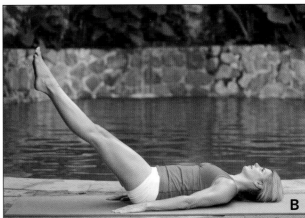

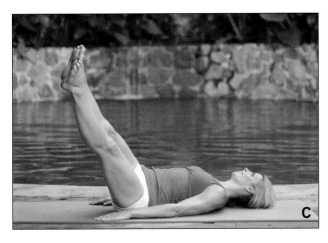

**POSITION 1:** Keeping your knees and ankles together, make a small circle with your legs to the right, letting your left hip come off the mat slightly (A).

**POSITION 2:** Circle your legs away from you (B).

**POSITION 3:** Complete the circle to the left. Reverse the direction—circle left and finish right for one complete circle (C). Do 10 to 12 reps.

## FABULOUS FORM TIPS

○ Don't lift your head or shoulders off the mat.

○ Keep your circles small so you can maintain good form until you get strong enough.

○ Don't separate your legs; squeeze your inner thighs to give you lots of power!

# **3** reach and twist with 3-pound ball

○○○○

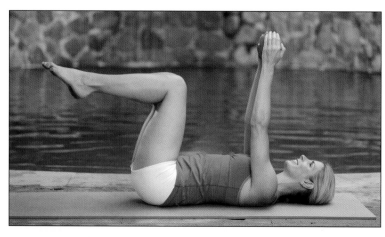

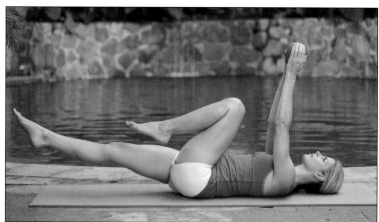

**STARTING POSITION:** Lie on your back with your knees bent at a 90-degree angle. Hold a 3-pound (1.5-kg) ball in your hands and straighten your arms over your nose, resting your head on the mat. Inhale in the starting position. Straighten your right leg so it's about nose level—toes in line with your nose— while your left knee remains near your chest.

## the payoff:
Takes your waist to a new skinny-level!

**sets -n- reps:** Do three sets of 10 to 12 reps.
**must-haves:** 3-pound (1.5-kg) ball

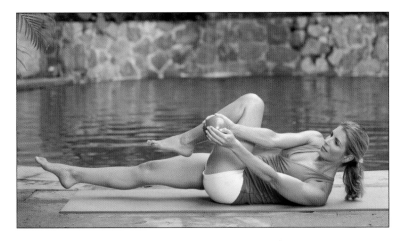

**POSITION 1:** Exhale to lift your head, neck, and shoulders off the ground, and twist to move the ball past your left knee, armpit to knee.

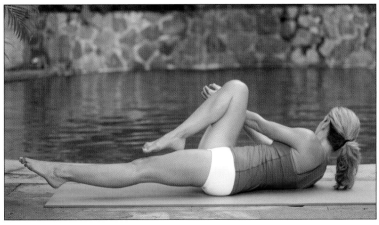

**POSITION 2:** Exhale to switch legs and twist to move the ball past your right knee, armpit to knee. Do 10 to 12 reps.

## FABULOUS FORM TIPS

○ Use your tummy muscles to lift, curl, and twist. The weighted ball creates extra work for your belly, so focus on good form.

○ Don't move from your neck—a big no-no! Not only can you hurt the delicate neck spine muscles, but you also won't be working your waist—so not sexy!

# **3** straight line side lifts

**sets -n- reps:** Do three sets of 10 to 12 reps.
**must-haves:** Nothing

○○○○

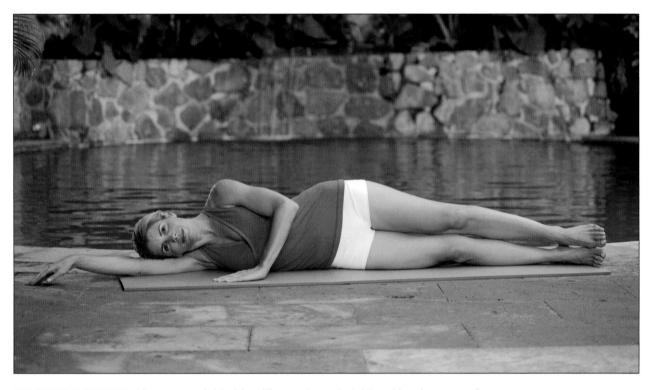

**STARTING POSITION:** Lie on your right side with your legs straight, ankles, knees, and hipbones stacked on top of one another, feet flexed and parallel. Straighten your right arm and lower your head to rest on it.

## the payoff:

Cinches your center!

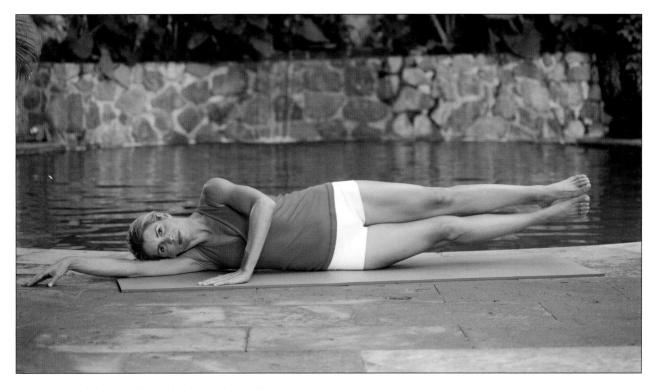

**POSITION 1:** Inhale to lift both of your legs off the ground and then exhale to lower your legs toward the floor, about 1 inch (2.5 cm) off the ground. Do 10 to 12 reps, and then switch sides.

## FABULOUS FORM TIPS

○ Don't strain in your lower back to lift your legs; engage your abs by lifting your belly button to your spine the whole time to protect your lower back.

○ Don't twist your body. Instead, imagine your body is between two pieces of glass.

○ Use your deep waist muscles to lift your legs. You should have a little space underneath your abs on the mat.

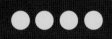

**WORKOUT 4:**

# super advanced

reach and twist with straight legs
(3-pound [1.5-kg] ball)

straight line side lifts
(3-pound [1.5-kg] ball)

windshield wiper legs
(isometric)

**THE PAYOFF:** Defines your lovely waist!

**TOTAL TIME:** 20 minutes

**HOW OFTEN:** By now, you should feel it (the tightening in your tummy) every time you work. Spend as much time as you want to scorch your love handles. Do this workout three times a week on nonconsecutive days.

★ **GETTING A WICKEDLY FLAT TUMMY,**
on page 15, offers more advice
for maximizing this workout.

# 4 reach and twist

○ ○ ○ ○

**sets -n- reps:** Do three sets of 10 to 12 reps.
**must-haves:** 3-pound (1.5-kg) ball

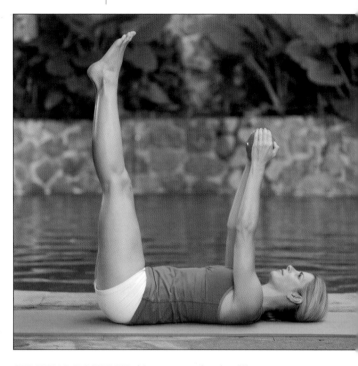

**STARTING POSITION:** Lie on your back with your legs straight, lengthening to the ceiling at a 90-degree angle or in line with your hipbones. Hold a 3-pound (1.5-kg) ball in your hands and then straighten your arms over your nose, resting your head on the mat. Inhale in the starting position.

## the payoff:

A money middle!

# with straight legs (3-pound [1.5-kg] ball)

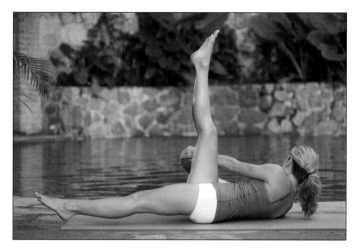

**POSITION 1:** Exhale to simultaneously straighten your right leg to the floor while your left leg lengthens to the ceiling and lift your head, neck, and shoulders off the ground to reach the ball past the outside of your left knee. Inhale to the starting position.

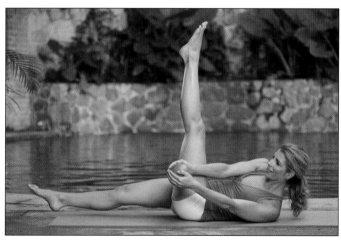

**POSITION 2:** Exhale to simultaneously straighten your left leg to the floor while your right leg lengthens to the ceiling and lift your head, neck, and shoulders off the ground to reach the ball past the outside of your right knee. Inhale to the starting position. Do 10 to 12 reps.

## FABULOUS FORM TIPS

○ Use your tummy muscles to lift, curl, and twist. The weighted ball creates extra work for your belly so focus on good form first.

○ Don't move from your neck—a big no-no! Not only can you hurt the delicate neck spine muscles, but you're also not working your waist—so not sexy!

○ Don't move fast; feel your waist whittle away as you work.

# 4 straight line side lifts (3-pound

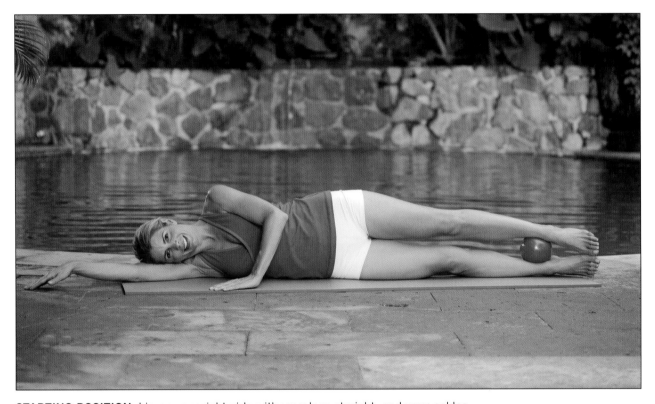

**STARTING POSITION:** Lie on your right side with your legs straight, and your ankles, knees, and hipbones stacked on top of one another, feet flexed and parallel. Place a 3-pound (1.5-kg) ball between your ankles. Straighten your right arm and lower your head to rest on it.

## the payoff:

Whittles your waist "way-away!"

# [1.5-kg] ball)

**sets -n- reps:** Do three sets of 10 to 12 reps.
**must-haves:** 3-pound (1.5-kg) ball

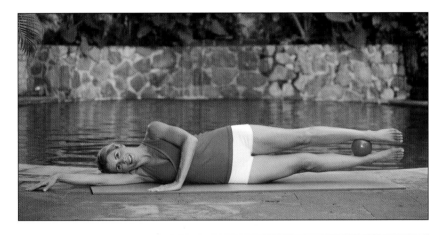

**POSITION 1:** Inhale to lift both of your legs off the ground and then exhale to lower your legs toward the floor, just about 1 inch (2.5 cm) off the ground. Do 10 to 12 reps, and then switch sides.

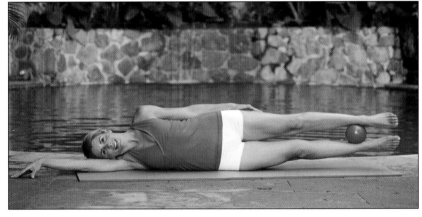

**POSITION 2:** Straighten your arm on your side. Repeat.

## FABULOUS FORM TIPS

❍ Don't strain your lower back to lift your legs. Instead, engage your abs by lifting your belly button to your spine to protect your lower back.

❍ Don't twist your body. Imagine your body is between two pieces of glass.

❍ Use your deep waist muscles to lift your legs. You should have a little space underneath your waist on the mat.

# **4** windshield wiper legs (isometric)

○○○○

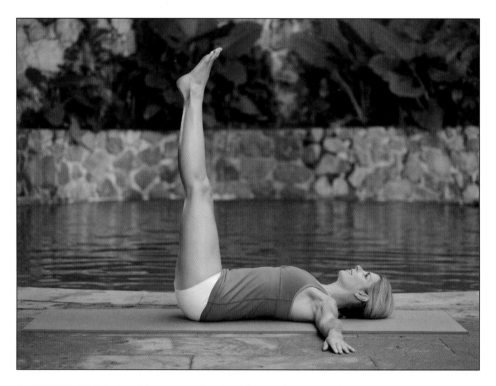

**STARTING POSITION:** Lie on your back with your legs straight, lengthening to the ceiling at a 90-degree angle or in line with your hipbones. Straighten your arms out to your sides so they form the letter T. Drop the back of your shoulders against the mat, and slide your shoulders away from your ears.

## **the payoff:**

Strengthens your waist stunning!

**sets -n- reps:** Do three sets of 10 to 12 reps.
**must-haves:** Nothing

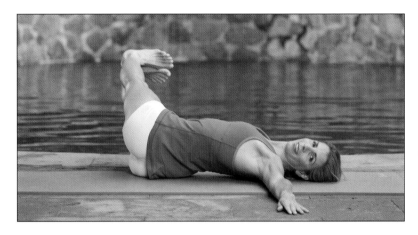

**POSITION 1:** Keeping your knees and ankles together, lower your legs to the right so your left hip comes off the mat. Don't rest your legs on the floor; hold 'em up to work your skinny waist. Hold this position for 5 to 10 seconds, and then exhale to the starting position.

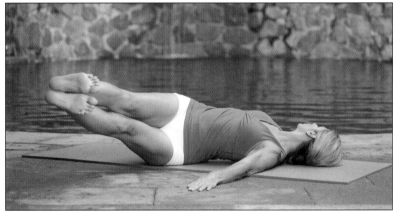

**POSITION 2:** Keeping your knees and ankles together, lower your legs to the left so your right hip comes off the mat. Don't rest your legs on the floor. Hold this position for 5 to 10 seconds, and then exhale to the starting position. Do *only* 5 reps on each side.

# FABULOUS FORM TIPS

❍ Don't lift your head or shoulders off the mat. Keep the movement small until you build enough strength in your deep obliques.

❍ Don't separate your legs. Squeeze your inner thighs to give you lots of power!

❍ Tighten your obliques like crazy to hold the isometric move, meaning no movement.

❍ If you feel lower back strain, try bending your knees.

❍ Fire up your waist muscles to bring your legs back into the starting position and move slowly with control to feel the contraction.

❍ Only lower your legs as low as your back allows.

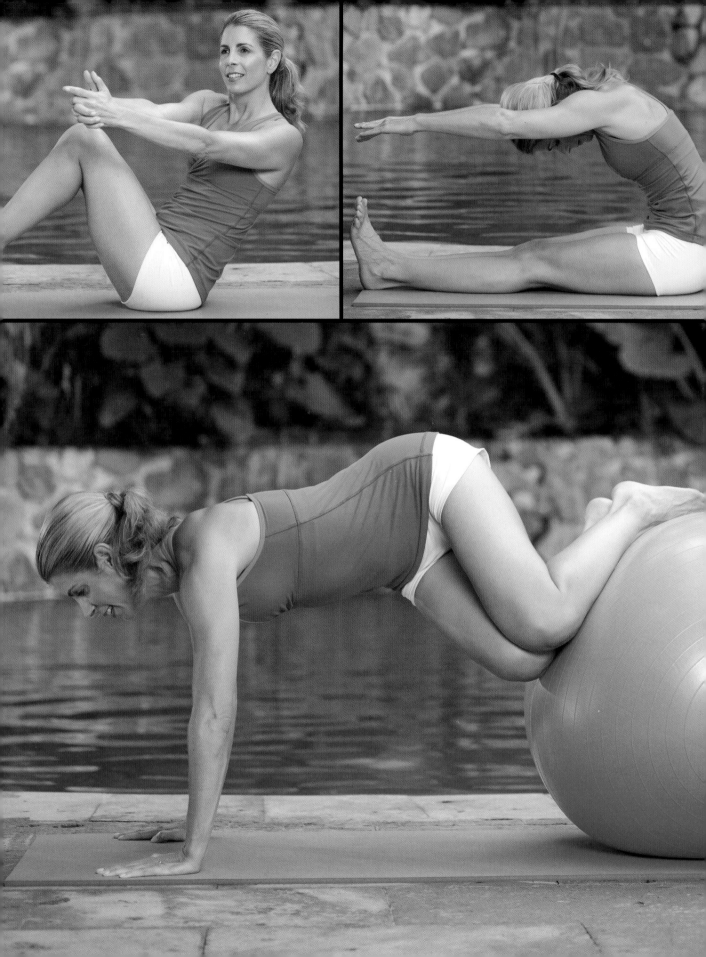

# chapter 3

# FAB ABS

| | | the payoff | total time | how often | sets -n- reps | must-haves |
|---|---|---|---|---|---|---|
| **WORKOUT 1:**<br>beginner<br><br>Front Plank<br>Roll Up<br>Teaser One | ○○○○ | Gives you a beautifully toned belly! | 15 to 20 minutes | Do this workout 3 times a week on non-consecutive days, such as Mon., Wed., and Fri. | Do three sets of 5 to 8 reps. | Nothing |
| **WORKOUT 2:**<br>intermediate<br><br>*Charlie's Angels* Abs<br>Side Plank<br>Plank on Ball | ○○○○ | Super-tones your tummy! | 15 to 20 minutes | Do this workout 3 times a week on non-consecutive days, such as Mon., Wed., and Fri. | Do three sets of 8 to 10 reps. | Stability ball |
| **WORKOUT 3:**<br>advanced<br><br>Reverse Curl-Plank on Ball<br>Front Plank with Twist<br>Teaser | ○○○○ | Takes you from paunchy to *abso* perfectly! | 15 to 20 minutes | Do this workout 3 times a week on non-consecutive days, such as Mon., Wed., and Fri. | Do three sets of 10 to 12 reps. | Stability ball |
| **WORKOUT 4:**<br>super advanced<br><br>Double Leg Lift with<br>  Knee to Chest Combo<br>Teaser with Leg Lifts<br>Plank on Ball with<br>  Knee to Chest Combo | ○○○○ | Gives you amazing, sexy-strong abs! | 15 to 20 minutes | Do this workout 3 times a week on non-consecutive days, such as Mon., Wed., and Fri. | Do three sets of as many as you can with good form! | Stability ball |

○●○○
**WORKOUT 1:**
# beginner
front plank
roll up
teaser one

---

**THE PAYOFF:**
## Gives you a beautifully toned belly!

---

**TOTAL TIME:** 15 to 20 minutes

**HOW OFTEN:** Spend two to four weeks strengthening your abs and focusing on finding a neutral pelvis to protect your lower back. Do this workout three times a week on nonconsecutive days.

★ **GETTING A WICKEDLY FLAT TUMMY,** on page 15, offers more advice for maximizing this workout.

# 1  front plank

○○○○

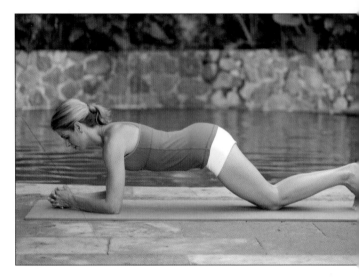

**STARTING POSITION:** Get on your knees and place your elbows directly under your shoulders, and interlace your fingers. With your toes curled under, place your heels together.

## the payoff:
A totally tight core!

**sets -n- reps:** Do three sets of 5 to 8 reps.

**must-haves:** Nothing

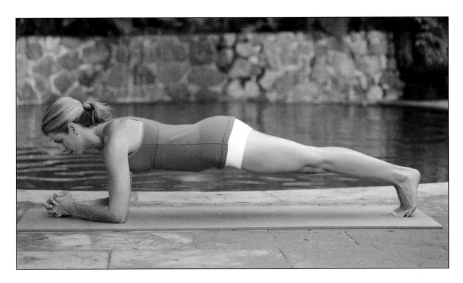

**POSITION 1:** Lift your legs, pelvis, and torso off the floor in one motion. Balance on your toes and elbows. Hold for 15 seconds.

# FABULOUS FORM TIPS

- ❍ Don't let your belly sag. Instead, gently lift your belly button to your spine to strengthen your abs and support your lower back.

- ❍ Don't lift your shoulders. Engage your back muscles by drawing your shoulders away from your ears.

- ❍ Don't drop your head—big no-no! Your head should be in line with your spine, always!

- ❍ Use your fanny. Don't lift it in the air but firm it up and squeeze your inner thighs—oh-so-much power lost if you don't use 'em!

# 1 roll up

○○○○

**sets -n- reps:** Do three sets of 5 to 8 reps.
**must-haves:** Nothing

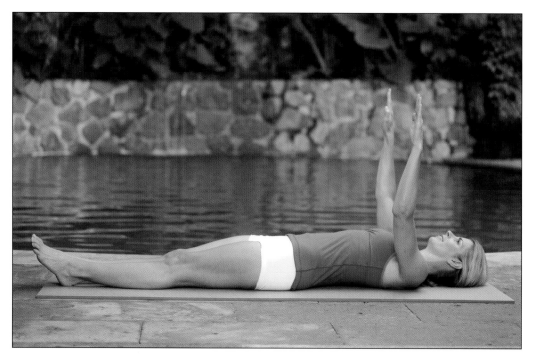

**STARTING POSITION:** Lie on your back with your legs straight. Straighten and lift your arms so your fingertips reach to the ceiling. Drop the back of your shoulders against the mat, and slide your shoulders away from your ears.

## the payoff:

Smooth out your rolls!

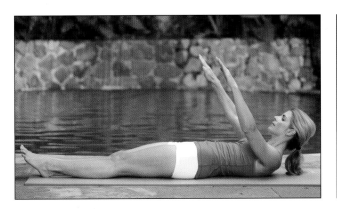

**POSITION 1:** Inhale to curl your chin to your chest, lifting the back of your shoulders off the mat to look between your arms. Keep your neck long.

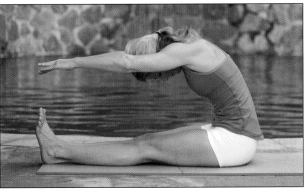

**POSITION 2:** Exhale to round over, belly button to your spine. Reach your fingers past your toes and flex your feet to stretch your hamstrings.

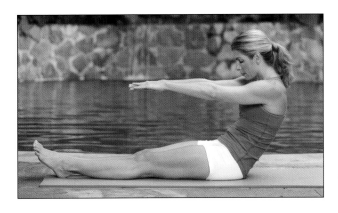

**POSITION 3:** Inhale to lift your pubic bone toward the ceiling, engaging your lower tummy. Exhale to roll down, bone by bone, to the starting position. Do 5 to 8 reps.

## FABULOUS FORM TIPS

- ❍ If you feel any lower back tension, start with your knees bent.

- ❍ Don't lift your shoulders to your ears; imagine a string from your armpits to your hips.

- ❍ Don't jerk up. If you can't roll up in a controlled motion, bend your knees and grab the backs of your thighs to help you.

- ❍ Don't plop down. Control is crucial, so try rolling down as you press your heels away from your hips.

- ❍ Squeeze your inner thighs. Imagine a rolled-up hand towel between your legs to work your inner thighs.

- ❍ Look at your belly to keep your head in line with your spine the whole time. Neck tension is so not sexy.

# 1 teaser one

**sets -n- reps:** Do three sets of 5 to 8 reps.
**must-haves:** Nothing

○○○○

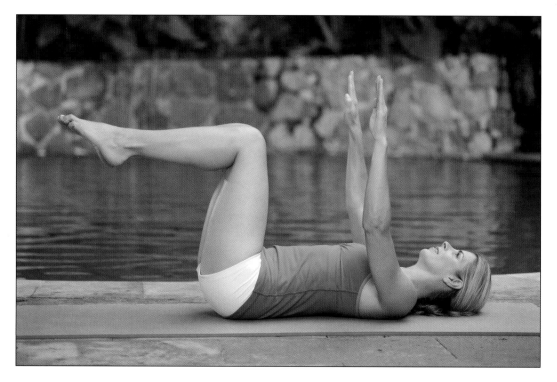

**STARTING POSITION:** Lie on your back with your knees bent at a 90-degree angle or directly in line with your hipbones. Your lower back should be flat on the floor, engaging your lower tummy muscles. Straighten your arms, lengthening your fingertips to the ceiling. Drop the back of your shoulders against the mat, and slide your shoulders down away from your ears.

## the payoff:

Tones all over belly!

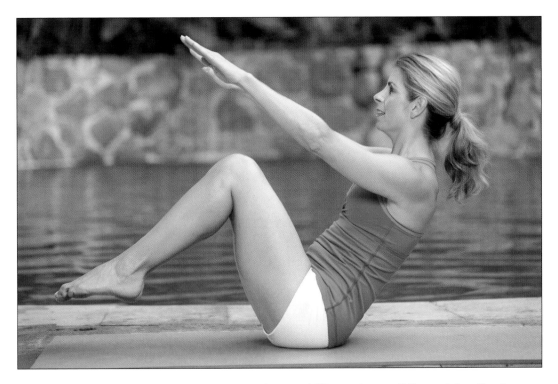

**POSITION 1:** Inhale to curl your chin to your chest and lift your torso off the mat, lengthening your fingertips past your knees. Exhale to tip your pubic bone, engaging your lower tummy, and roll down so you feel each bone on the mat. Do 5 to 8 reps.

## FABULOUS FORM TIPS

❍ Don't jerk up. Instead, gently curl your chin to peel your spine off the mat. If you can't come up, hold your thighs to help you—just don't strain.

❍ Don't lift your shoulders; engage your back muscles by drawing your shoulders away from your ears.

❍ Use your abs as you roll down. You don't want to miss out on the yummy tummy work!

**WORKOUT 2:**
# intermediate

*charlie's angels* abs
side plank
plank on ball

---

**THE PAYOFF:**
## Super-tones your tummy!

---

**TOTAL TIME:** 15 to 20 minutes

**HOW OFTEN:** Spend two to four weeks strengthening your abs. Now I want you to actually feel the tightening in your tummy. Do this workout three times a week on nonconsecutive days.

★ **GETTING A WICKEDLY FLAT TUMMY,**
**on page 15, offers more advice**
**for maximizing this workout.**

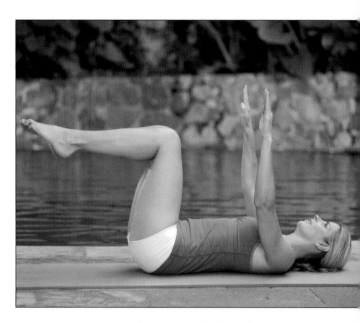

**STARTING POSITION:** Lie on your back with your knees bent at a 90-degree angle or directly in line with your hipbones. Your lower back should be flat on the floor, engaging your lower tummy muscles. Straighten your arms, raising your fingertips to the ceiling. Drop the back of your shoulders against the mat, and slide your shoulders away from your ears.

## the payoff:
Sculpts a marvelous midsection!

# abs

**sets -n- reps:** Do three sets of 8 to 10 reps.
**must-haves:** Nothing

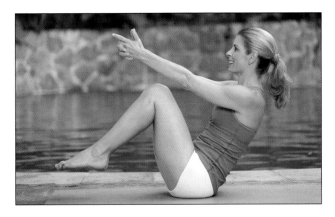

**POSITION 1:** Inhale to curl your chin to your chest and lift your torso off the mat. Clasp your hands, and make a gun like one of *Charlie's Angels* with your hands—ha!

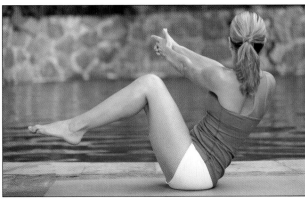

**POSITION 2:** Inhale to lengthen your spine and then slowly twist to the right.

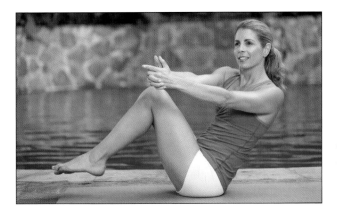

**POSITION 3:** Inhale to position 1 and then slowly twist to the left. Remember, you're twisting from the bottom rib while in the Teaser position. Do three *Charlie's Angels* and then roll down, feeling every bone touching the mat. Do 8 to 10 reps.

## FABULOUS FORM TIPS

○ Don't jerk up. Gently curl your chin to peel your spine off the mat. If you can't come up, hold your thighs to help you—just don't strain.

○ Don't lift your shoulders. Engage your back muscles by drawing your shoulders away from your ears.

○ Twist from your bottom ribs and stay stable in your hips as you twist to get the killer waist work.

○ Use your abs as you roll down. You don't want to miss out on the yummy tummy work!

# **2** side plank

○○○○

**sets -n- reps:** Do three sets of 8 to 10 reps.
**must-haves:** Nothing

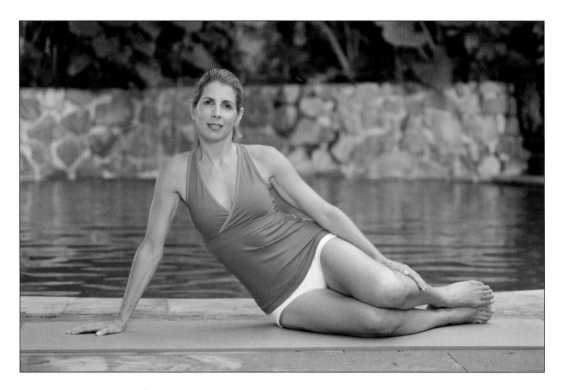

**STARTING POSITION:** Sit on your right side with your knees slightly pulled into your body, stacking your knees on top of one another. Place your right hand on the floor directly under your right shoulder.

## the payoff:

Whittles your waist!

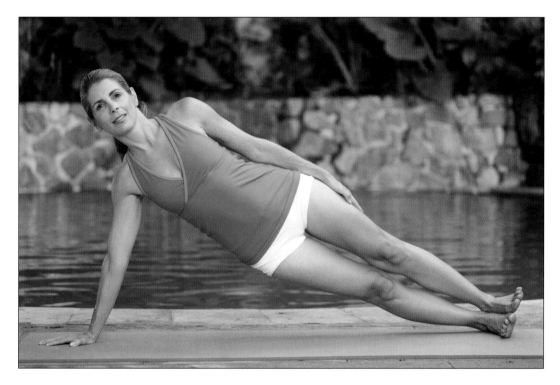

**POSITION 1.** Lift your torso, hips, and legs off the floor in one motion. Balance on your right hand and on the right leading edge of your foot, stacking your feet on top of one another. Repeat three times, holding for 15 seconds, and then switch sides.

## FABULOUS FORM TIPS

○ Don't drop your torso in the middle. Focus on your breath work to engage and lift your waist muscles to the ceiling.

○ Don't hang in your wrist. Your wrist should line up under your shoulder and lift, lift, lift!

# **2** plank on ball

**sets -n- reps:** Do three sets of 8 to 10 reps.
**must-haves:** Stability ball

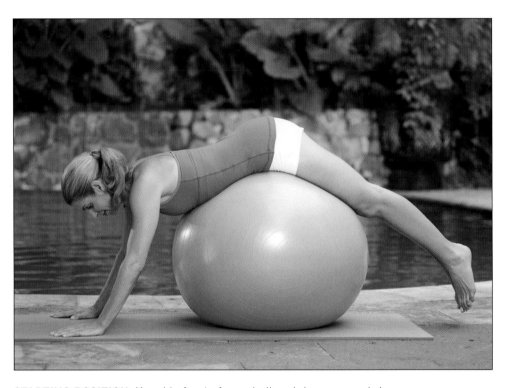

**STARTING POSITION:** Kneel in front of your ball and drape your abdomen and hips over the ball. Place your hands on the floor in front of the ball.

## the payoff:

Gives you a flat tummy—and strong back!

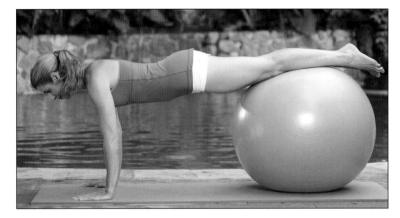

**POSITION 1:** Walk your hands out until the ball rolls toward your knees. Once you're stable, hold for 30 seconds as your body remains solid and straight, with a slight arch. Focus on lifting your belly button to your spine the whole time so you get the much-desired lower belly work. Squeeze your thighs for inner thigh power.

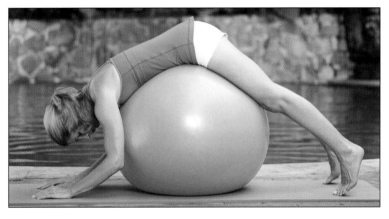

**POSITION 2:** Drape your body over the ball to stretch your lower back.

## FABULOUS FORM TIPS

❍ Don't let your lower belly sag. If you feel pressure in your lower back, make sure your hips are not below the ball and lift your belly button to your spine with every deep exhalation.

❍ Contract your inner thighs for extra power. Ladies, it works!

❍ Don't do this exercise if you have a shoulder or neck injury.

❍ Don't open your arms too wide. Instead, align your wrists directly under your shoulders while your shoulder blades slide down your back to create shoulder stability and work your upper back muscles. To alleviate wrist pain, consider gripping a pair of dumbbell weights to elevate your wrists in a neutral position.

❍ Don't drop your head. Instead, lengthen from the top of your head and gaze at the floor.

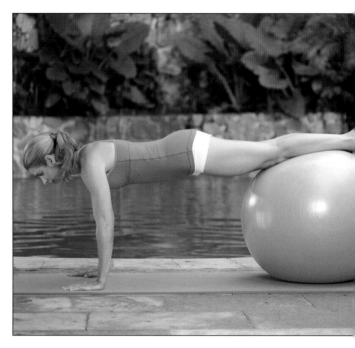

**STARTING POSITION:** Kneel in front of your ball and drape your abdomen and hips over the ball. Place your hands on the floor in front of the ball. Walk your hands out until the ball rolls toward your knees.

● ● ● ○

**WORKOUT 3:**
# advanced

reverse curl-plank on ball
front plank with twist
teaser

---

**THE PAYOFF:**
## Takes you from paunchy to *abso* perfectly!

---

**TOTAL TIME:** 15 to 20 minutes

**HOW OFTEN:** By now, you should be sweating it out. This workout is mega-hard! Spend two to four weeks to get your abs smoking hot. Do this workout three times a week on nonconsecutive days.

★ **GETTING A WICKEDLY FLAT TUMMY,**
on page 15, offers more advice
for maximizing this workout.

## the payoff:
Causes outbreak of ab-envy!

# plank on ball

**sets -n- reps:** Do three sets of 10 to 12 reps.
**must-haves:** Stability ball

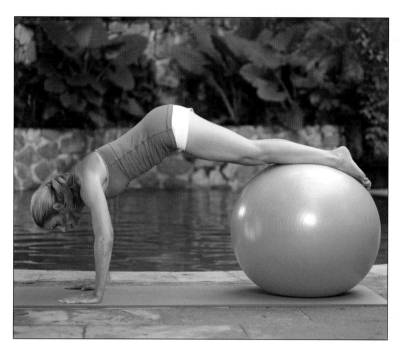

**POSITION 1:** When you're stable, deeply contract from your sweet spot to lift your hips an inch or so. The focus is on tightening your lower tummy with every lift, pulsing to keep the ab work intense. Do 10 to 12 reps. Drape your body over the ball to stretch your lower back.

## FABULOUS FORM TIPS

○ Don't let your lower belly sag. If you feel pressure in your lower back, make sure your hips are not below the ball and lift your belly button to your spine with every deep exhalation.

○ Don't lift your heiny too high. Use your inner thighs for extra strength.

○ Don't do this exercise if you have a shoulder or neck injury.

○ Don't open your arms too wide. Align your wrists directly under your shoulders while your shoulder blades slide down your back to create shoulder stability and work your upper back muscles.

○ Don't drop your head. Lengthen from the top of your head and gaze at the floor.

# **3** front plank with twist

○○○○

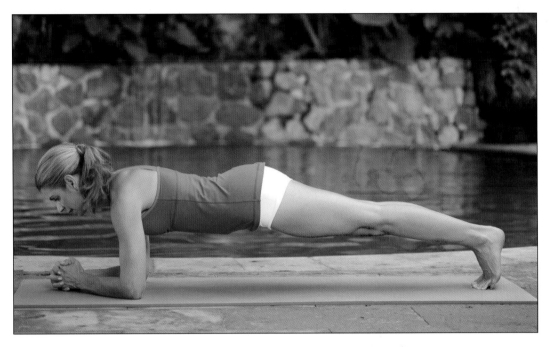

**STARTING POSITION:** Get on your knees, place your elbows directly under your shoulders, and interlace your fingers. With your toes curled under, place your heels together. Inhale to lift your legs, pelvis, and torso off the floor in one motion into a plank postion.

## **the payoff:**

Super slims your waist!

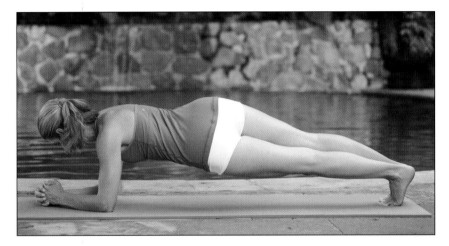

**POSITION 1:** Exhale to twist ever so slightly to the right from your waist *only*. You really need to fire up your waist muscles to isolate the work. Inhale to the starting position.

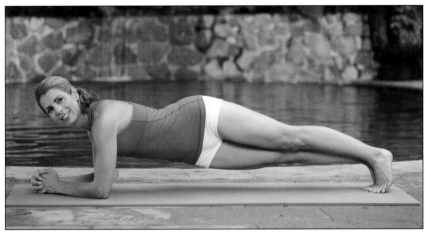

**POSITION 2:** Exhale to twist ever so slightly to the left from your waist only. Do 10 to 12 reps.

## FABULOUS FORM TIPS

❍ Don't let your belly sag. Instead, gently lift your belly button to your spine to strengthen your abs and support your lower back.

❍ Don't lift your shoulders; engage your back muscles by drawing your shoulders away from your ears.

❍ Don't drop you head—big no-no! Your head should be in line with your spine, always!

❍ Move from your waist only. Don't move your entire body, otherwise you'll miss out on the delicious waist work.

# **3** teaser

**sets -n- reps:** Do three sets of 10 to 12 reps.
**must-haves:** Nothing

○○○○

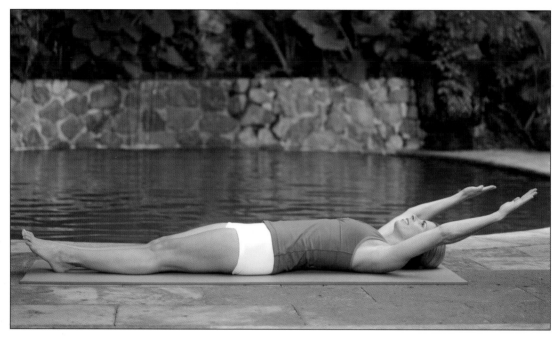

**STARTING POSITION:** Lie on your back with your legs straight on the mat. Straighten your arms over your head. Engage your tummy now!

## the payoff:

Gives you amazing all-over abs!

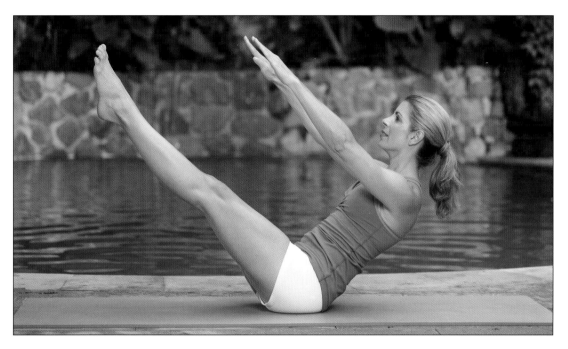

**POSITION 1:** Inhale to curl your chin to your chest and lift your torso and legs off the mat simultaneously, lengthening your fingertips to your toes. You're making a V with your body. Exhale to tip your pubic bone, engaging your lower tummy, and roll down so you feel each bone on the mat. Do 10 to 12 reps.

## FABULOUS FORM TIPS

○ Don't jerk up. Instead, engage your lower tummy to come up and roll down.

○ Exhale deeply to melt each bone of your spine down to the mat.

○ Use your abs to hold the Teaser, keeping your belly button to your spine the whole time.

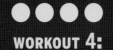

WORKOUT 4:

# super advanced

double leg lift with knee
to chest combo

teaser with leg lifts

plank on ball with knee
to chest combo

---

**THE PAYOFF:**

## Gives you amazing, sexy-strong abs!

**TOTAL TIME:** 15 to 20 minutes

**HOW OFTEN:** By now, your tummy is working at full throttle! Spend two to four weeks to keep your abs looking great. Do this workout three times a week on nonconsecutive days.

★ **GETTING A WICKEDLY FLAT TUMMY,**
on page 15, offers more advice
for maximizing this workout.

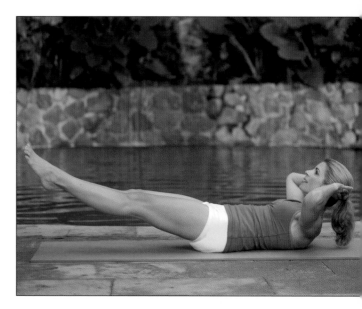

**STARTING POSITION:** Lie on your back with your legs straight, lengthening to the ceiling at a 90-degree angle or in line with your hipbones. Lift your head, neck, and shoulders off the ground. Inhale to straighten your legs so they're about nose level.

## the payoff:

Builds muscle and tones all
your tummy muscles

# with knee to chest combo

**sets -n- reps:** Do three sets of as many as you can with good form!

**must-haves:** Nothing

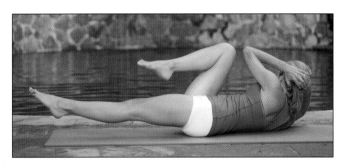

**POSITION 1:** Exhale to bring your right knee to your left elbow. Lift and twist from your bottom rib so you feel the work in your waist.

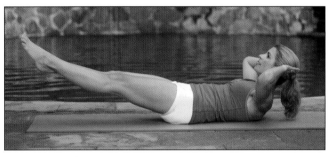

**POSITION 2:** Inhale to the starting position.

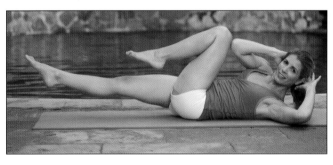

**POSITION 3:** Exhale to bring your left knee to your right elbow. Lift and twist from your bottom rib so you feel the work in your waist. Do 10 to 12 reps.

## FABULOUS FORM TIPS

❍ Use your lower tummy muscles to stabilize your body as you bring your knee into your elbow.

❍ Keep your legs in line with your nose the whole time, never relaxing your abs until all reps are complete!

❍ Feel the sweet spot. This is a super-advanced exercise, so do what you can do with good form.

# **4** teaser with leg lifts

**sets -n- reps:** Do three sets of as many as you can with good form!

**must-haves:** Nothing

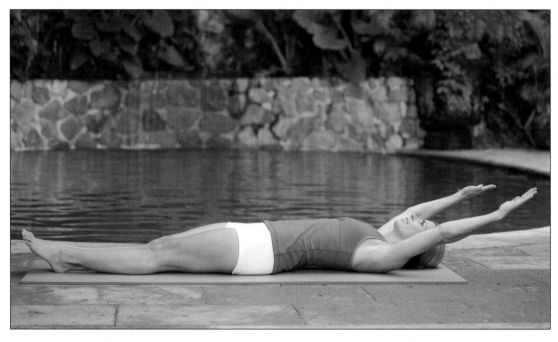

**STARTING POSITION:** Lie on your back with your legs straight on the mat. Straighten your arms over your head. Engage your tummy now!

## the payoff:

Sculpts your tummy sexy-flat!

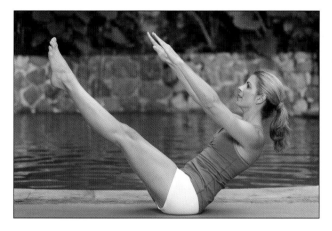

**POSITION 1:** Inhale to curl your chin to your chest and lift your arms and legs off the mat, lengthening your fingertips to your toes. You're making a V, or a Teaser, with your body.

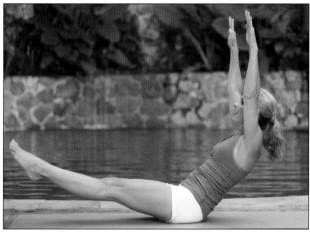

**POSITION 2:** As you hold the Teaser, lower your legs to the floor, exhale, and then lift your legs up. Do three leg lifts and then exhale to tip your pubic bone, engaging your lower tummy, and roll down so you feel each bone on the mat. Do 10 to 12 reps.

## FABULOUS FORM TIPS

○ Don't jerk up. Engage your lower tummy to come up and roll down.

○ Exhale deeply to melt each bone of your spine down to the mat.

○ Use your abs to lower and lift your legs. Wow, major belly work! Focus on sinking your belly button to your spine every time you lower and lift your legs.

# **4** plank on ball with knee to chest

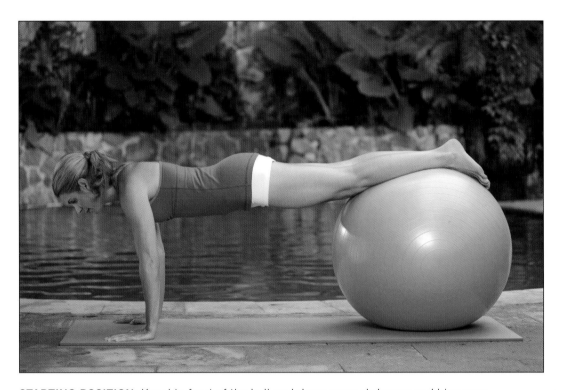

**STARTING POSITION:** Kneel in front of the ball and drape your abdomen and hips over the ball. Place your hands on the floor in front of the ball. Walk your hands out until the ball rolls toward your knees.

## the payoff:

Gives you a teeny waist and strong back!

# combo

**sets -n- reps:** Do three sets of as many as you can with good form!

**must-haves:** Stability ball

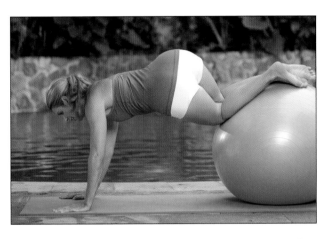

**POSITION 1:** Once you're stable, bend your knees and roll the ball to the right, feeling the twist in your waist.

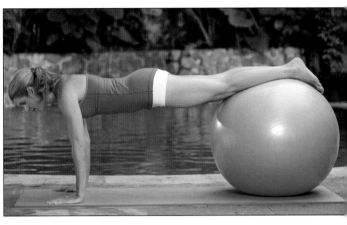

**POSITION 2:** Straighten your legs into the plank position. Focus on lifting your belly button to your spine the whole time so you get the much-desired lower belly work. Squeeze your thighs for inner thigh power.

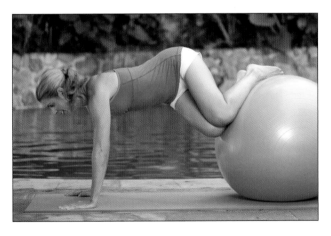

**POSITION 3:** Once you're stable, bend your knees and roll the ball to the left, feeling the twist in your waist. Drape over the ball to stretch your lower back. Do 10 to 12 reps.

## FABULOUS FORM TIPS

○ Don't let your lower belly sag. If you feel pressure in your lower back, make sure your hips are not below the ball and lift your belly button to your spine with every deep exhalation.

○ Don't do this exercise if you have a shoulder or neck injury.

○ Don't open your arms too wide. Align your wrists directly under your shoulders.

○ Don't drop your head. Lengthen from the top of your head and gaze at the floor.

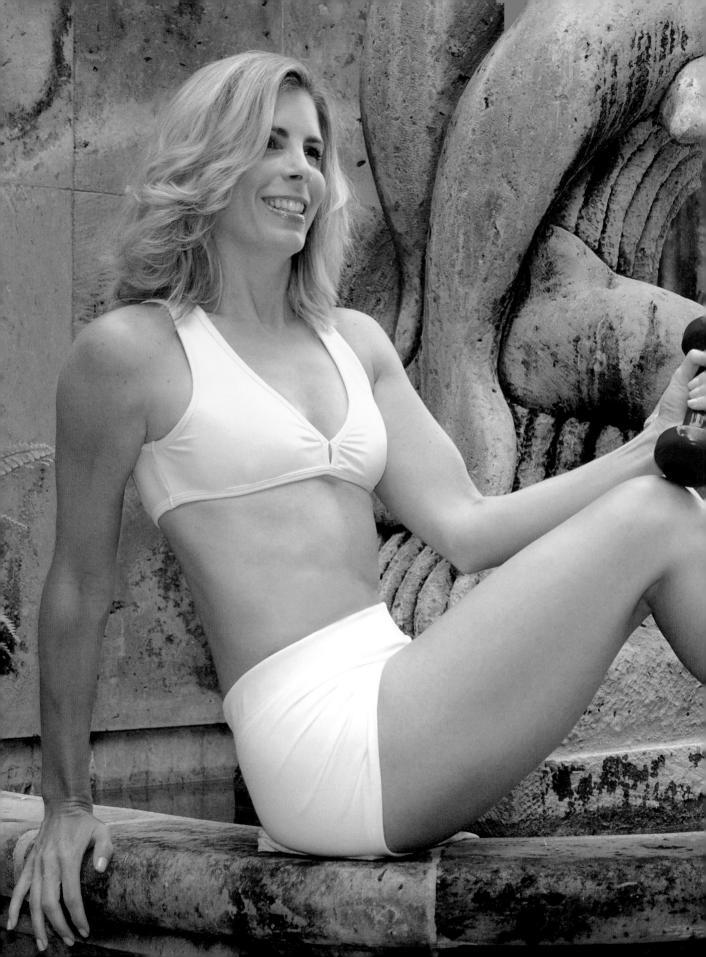

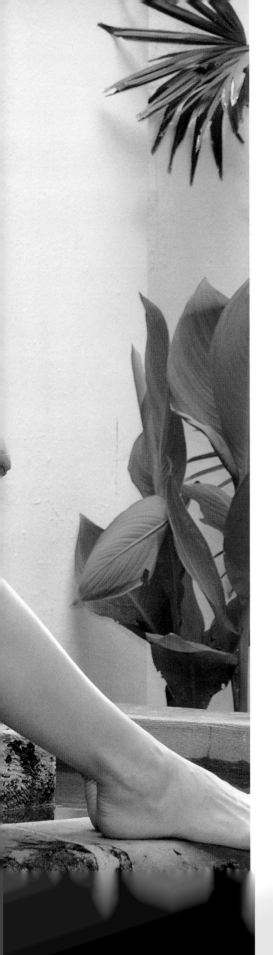

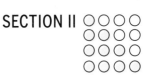

# The Best Lower Body Workouts

### fall in love with your body-hugging jeans!

**At last**—your best dream-jean body ever! Whether you want to shed several pounds or sculpt yourself gorgeous (or both!), the terrific toners, cardio blast, and eating tips in this section will help you wipe out the lumps on your legs and bumps on your booty.

Now, get ready for tons of fun in the workouts in the next four chapters.

**CHAPTER 4:** Bodacious Booty

**CHAPTER 5:** Slimtastic Outer Thighs

**CHAPTER 6:** Slimtastic Inner Thighs

**CHAPTER 7:** Cankles, Begone!

You'll fit into your body huggers in no time. Keep going, gorgeous!

# Melt Inches with Cardio

Zap calories and fight flab with a 50-minute sweat session on the treadmill. To lose a jaw-dropping pants size, you'll do two of my favorite super-effective treadmill workouts—incline treadmill to target your booty and multi-walking, in which you'll walk backward and sideways to target your inner and outer thighs.

Here's a warning: changing directions on the treadmill is a little tricky, so be careful. Reduce the speed before you turn directions, place your feet on the outer sides for stability before moving, and hold the handrails at all times.

If you don't have a gym membership or get bored with treadmills, you can do an incline work-out outside. Just find a hill or some school bleach-ers to get your rear in gear! Likewise, if you don't like the treadmill, the stair-stepper is best for your butt and legs. Pick your workout and do this cardio work four times a week.

## Incline Workout

Do this workout on the treadmill, a hill, or bleachers.

**INTERVAL ONE**
**2 minutes:** Warm up by walking 3.5 mph, no grade
**6 minutes:** Walk 4 mph, with a 5 percent incline. (You can hold a conversation, but it should be breathy!)
**2 minutes:** Walk 3.8 to 4.0 mph with a 10 percent incline. (Break-a-sweat pace: It should be hard to complete your sentences.)

**INTERVAL TWO**
**8 minutes:** Walk 4 mph, with a 5 percent incline
**2 minutes:** Walk 3.8 to 4.0 mph with a 10 percent incline

**INTERVAL THREE**
**8 minutes:** Walk 4 mph, with a 5 percent incline
**2 minutes:** Walk 3.8 to 4.0 mph with a 10 percent incline

**INTERVAL FOUR**
**8 minutes:** Walk 4 mph, with a 5 percent incline
**2 minutes:** Walk 3.8 to 4.0 mph with a 10 percent incline

**INTERVAL FIVE**
**6 minutes:** Walk 4 mph, with a 5 percent incline
**2 minutes:** Walk 3.8 to 4.0 mph with a 10 percent incline
**Cool down:** Walk 2 minutes at 3.2 to 3.5 mph, no grade

Also, If you can stay at a 10 percent incline for longer than 2 minutes in any of these intervals, go for it!

# Multi-Walking Workout

Try walking backward and sideways in the following steps, on the treadmill or on a track.

### INTERVAL ONE
**2 minutes:** Warm up by walking 3.5 mph, no grade
**5 minutes:** Walk facing front 3.8 to 4.0 mph, no grade
**1 minute:** Walk backward at 3.2 to 3.5 mph, no grade. (Sit deep in your thighs, press through your heels, and hold the handrails.)
**1 minute:** Walk sideways/squatting (right side) 1.8 to 2.0 mph, no grade. (Push off the leading foot to work your inner thighs and hold the handrails.)
**1 minute:** Walk sideways/squatting (left side) 1.8 to 2.0 mph, no grade. (Push off the leading foot to work your inner thighs and hold the handrail.)

### INTERVAL TWO
**7 minutes:** Walk facing front 3.8 to 4.0 mph, no grade
**1 minute:** Walk backward 3.2 to 3.5 mph, no grade
**1 minute:** Walk sideways/squatting (right side) 1.8 to 2.0 mph, no grade
**1 minute:** Walk sideways/squatting (left side) 1.8 to 2.0 mph, no grade

### INTERVAL THREE
**7 minutes:** Walk facing front 3.8 to 4.0 mph, no grade
**1 minute:** Walk backward 3.2 to 3.5 mph, no grade
**1 minute:** Walk sideways/squatting (right side) 1.8 to 2.0 mph, no grade
**1 minute:** Walk sideways/squatting (left side) 1.8 to 2.0 mph, no grade

### INTERVAL FOUR
**7 minutes:** Walk facing front 3.8 to 4.0 mph, no grade
**1 minute:** Walk backward 3.2 to 3.5 mph, no grade
**1 minute:** Walk sideways/squatting (right side) 1.8 to 2.0 mph, no grade
**1 minute:** Walk sideways/squatting (left side) 1.8 to 2.0 mph, no grade

### INTERVAL FIVE
**5 minutes:** Walk facing front 3.8 to 4.0 mph, no grade
**1 minute:** Walk backward 3.2 to 3.5 mph, no grade
**1 minute:** Walk sideways/squatting (right side) 1.8 to 2.0 mph, no grade
**1 minute:** Walk sideways/squatting (left side) 1.8 to 2.0 mph, no grade
**2 minutes:** Cool down by walking 3.5 mph, no grade

Here's a warning: take your time turning backward and sideways on the treadmill. Follow these steps.

- Input the prescribed mph.
- Hold the handrails.
- Put your feet on the outer sides of the treadmill for stability.
- Turn around, placing your feet back on the outer sides of the treadmill.
- Once you're steady, start walking on the treadmill again.

Always turn to the front first to input the prescribed mph setting and then get into position for the prescribed time. Don't fret if you can't complete the prescribed exercise time. I'm giving you minutes based on how I work out. In other words, make it a goal and before long you'll become a pro at moving on the treadmill—and it gets your gams gorgeous, too!

# Getting to Know Your Muscles

Here's a chance to get to know your muscles that are going to shape your look from behind.

The **gluteals**, or glutes, are a group of muscles that make or break your backside. The gluteus maximus is the largest muscle in your body, generating lots of power for you to sit, stand, or run. Beneath it are a pair of deep, fanlike muscles that also provide hip stability—the gluteus medius, which travels along your outer thigh, and the gluteus minimus, which sits a little higher up on the hip. These exercises do target your maximus, but you'll get some work for all of your glutes in these exercises.

Your **hamstrings**, or hams, are the muscles of the upper back of the leg, originating on your butt bones, which is why it's hard to work your butt without calling them into play. Together these muscles—biceps femoris, semitendinosus, and semimembranosus—run down the backs of your legs, attaching on the outside of your knees, and have different roles in your body. These muscles help stabilize your hips and joints so you can bend over or kick a ball without getting injured.

Your **spinal erectors**, or back muscles, run the length of your spine, all the way to the base of your skull. These muscles, when strong, keep your spine healthy and flexible, and your posture perfect.

On the front side of your legs are your **quadriceps**, or quads, meaning these four muscles: rectus femoris, vastus lateralis, vastus medialis, and vastus intermedius. Similar to your hamstrings, these muscles originate high in the hips and run down the front thigh, attaching in a variety of places below the knee. Strong quads help support your knee (especially as you run) and literally help you sit, stand, and walk. Together, the hams and quads propel you forward—and keep your body in motion.

In chapter 5 the focus is on the outer thigh, or the aforementioned **gluteus medius and minimus**. These muscles, along with other deep hip rotators, help stabilize your hips, keeping you balanced and preventing you from tipping over. Collectively, these muscles are called your abductors, because they move your leg away from your body.

We attack the inside of your thighs in chapter 6—a group of muscles, known as your **adductors**. Individually, the inner thigh muscles are the adductors magnus, brevis, and longus; the gracillis; and the pectineus. They pull your legs together and create slimness in your thighs. Each adductor plays a different role in your body, but they, too, help stabilize your hips when you walk, run, stand, climb, and lunge.

Your calves primarily consist of two muscles, the **gastrocnemius** and the **soleus.** The gastrocnemius originates on your lower thighbone, just above your knee, while the soleus sits lower and a little deeper than your gastrocnemius.

Both muscles attach to the Achilles tendon, which attaches to your heel bone. When these muscles contract, you lift up on your tiptoes.

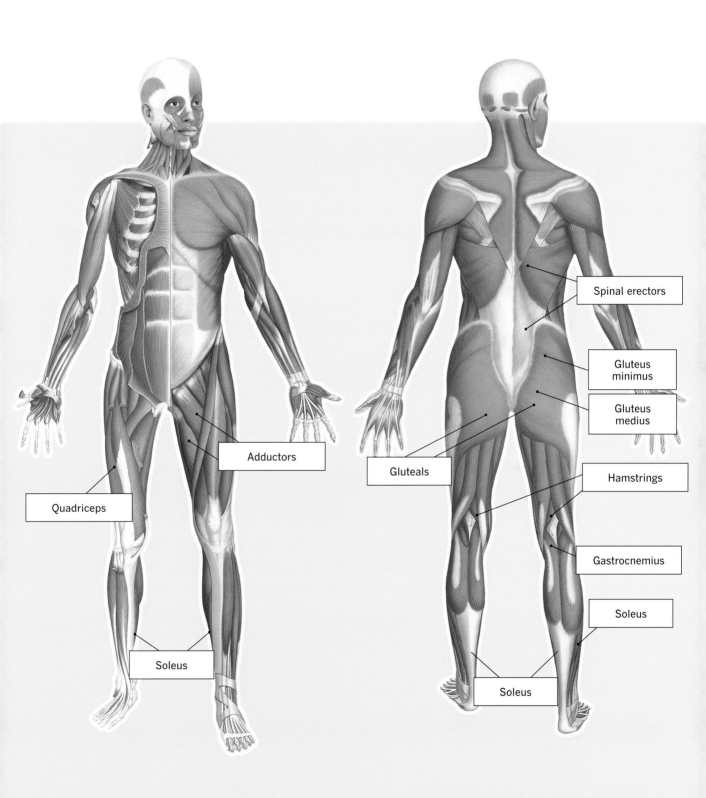

Spinal erectors

Gluteus minimus

Gluteus medius

Adductors

Hamstrings

Gluteals

Quadriceps

Gastrocnemius

Soleus

Soleus

Soleus

# Getting the Most Out of Your Workouts

## booty focus

To maintain the focus on your bum, keep in mind the following form tips in each booty exercise.

- **ENGAGE, SQUEEZE, AND FOCUS.** If you do nothing else, do this: in every butt exercise, you must tighten your booty so it's rock hard, because that's how great butts are made!

- **PENCIL IN BUTT CHEEKS.** Good form is a must. To avoid overdoing it with a pelvic tilt—so not sexy because it gives you a flat heiny—squeeze your bum together as if holding a pencil between your butt cheeks. (See page 11 to check out the pelvic tilt.)

- **WORK YOUR UNDERBUTT.** Hands down, your best weapon against the droopy area underneath your panties is a deadlift. But you must do your part and focus, squeeze, and tighten to give this area a little lift!

- **BURN, BOOTY, BURN.** Low weight means more reps, so go for the burn. (Yes, seriously, I haven't lost a student yet from booty overkill.)

- **PROTECT YOUR LOWER BACK.** To work safely and protect your lower back, lift your belly button to your spine the whole time to engage your tummy muscles.

## RESIZE YOUR THIGHS

The workouts for your thighs in chapter 5 and 6 go from out to in! Note that I start all exercises on your right side. Do all of the exercises (reps and all) on your right side, and then flip over to your left side to complete one set (unless I state otherwise). Then repeat the entire workout again to complete your second set and so forth until you do all three sets. For killer thighs, follow these alignment tips.

★ **Stack your hips.** Make sure your hips are even, stacked on top of one another at all times. Keeping good form is key to isolating your outer thighs and protecting your lower back.

★ **Use your abs.** To help keep your hips stable, engage your abs, lifting your belly button to your spine the whole time.

★ **Relax your neck.** No need to stress your neck and shoulders as you lose inches! Rest your head on your arm and focus on nothing else but heating up your thighs.

★ **Feel the burn.** Light weights mean more reps because you need to stimulate the muscle to the point of fatigue. Think slimtastic!

★ **Squeeze your thighs.** Don't haphazardly move your legs. Instead, laser-focus on your trouble zones to fully engage. I promise, you'll see and feel the difference.

# a guide to filling up and slimming down

Stop counting calories and start eating the right amount of precious nutrients. To lose those unwanted pounds, think small. A serving size isn't much, but you can still fill up by eating a variety of foods with lots of color (think crudités) on your plate every day. The goods news is that you won't have to kiss your sweets goodbye. Here's a sample food day.

○ **ONE SMALL SWEET,** such as ½ cup (125 g) of frozen yogurt or three small squares of dark chocolate

○ **TWO HEART-HEALTHY FATS,** such as 1 tablespoon (15 ml) of olive or canola oil or a small handful of walnuts (the size of the palm of your hand)

○ **TWO SERVINGS OF LEAN MEAT,** each the size of a deck of cards

○ **THREE SERVINGS OF LOW- OR NONFAT DAIRY PRODUCTS,** such as 4 ounces (125 g) of yogurt

○ **FIVE GRITTY GRAINS,** such as ½ cup (90 g) of cooked oatmeal, ½ cup (90 g) of a multigrain cereal, or 1 slice of multigrain bread. Eat them early, too—for breakfast or lunch—and then eat little to no carbs for dinner.

○ **TEN SERVINGS OF MIXED LEAFY GREENS AND FRUIT,** such as a small apple, 1 cup (30 g) of mixed greens, or ½ cup (75 g) of blueberries. Don't fret; this is easier than it sounds. For example, a healthy spinach salad with a few different veggies (and maybe some nuts or a little cheese for flavor) could just about get you there!

## SHAPE YOUR ANKLES

The workouts in chapter 7 focus on your calves. Although they are quite simple to do, you should keep in mind the following tips to isolate your calves.

★ When your toes are parallel, you're building good overall strength in your calves, which is important for optimal foot placement—and good posture, too.

★ When your toes point in, you're strengthening and shaping your outer calves.

★ When your toes point out, you're strengthening and shaping your inner calves.

★ As you lift up, engage your abs to help you balance.

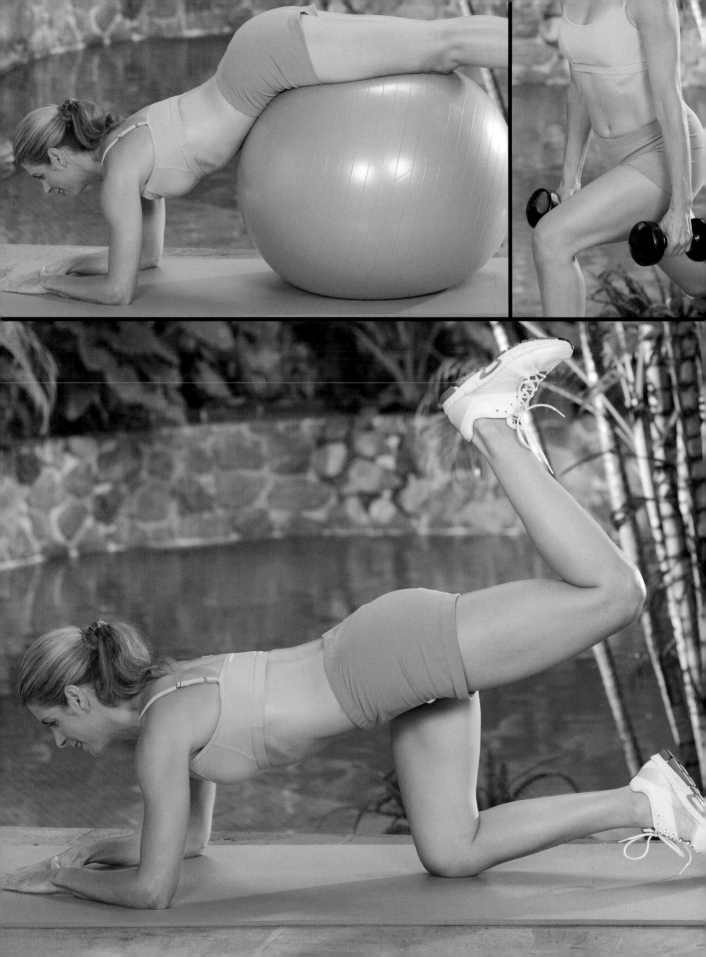

chapter 4

# BODACIOUS BOOTY

| | | the payoff | total time | how often | sets -n- reps | must-haves |
|---|---|---|---|---|---|---|
| **WORKOUT 1:**<br>beginner<br><br>Squat with Dumbbells<br>Deadlift with Dumbbells<br>Booty Hydrant | ○○○○ | Gets you bootyluscious—and sexy cheeky! | 15 to 20 minutes | Do this workout 3 times a week on non-consecutive days, such as Mon., Wed., and Fri. | Do three sets of 15 to 20 reps. | A pair of 10- to 15-pound (4.5- to 7-kg) dumbbells |
| **WORKOUT 2:**<br>intermediate<br><br>Froggy on Big Ball<br>Lateral Squat with Dumbbell<br>Leg Lifts on Ball | ○○○○ | Gives you goddess-worthy, grabbable glutes! | 15 to 20 minutes | Do this workout 3 times a week on non-consecutive days, such as Mon., Wed., and Fri. | Do three sets of 15 to 25 reps. | A pair of 8- to 15-pound (3.5- to 7-kg) dumbbells and a large exercise ball |
| **WORKOUT 3:**<br>advanced<br><br>Walking Lunges<br>Booty Hydrant with<br> 3-pound (1.5-kg) Ball<br>Plié Squat | ○○○○ | Kicks your underbutt! | 15 to 20 minutes | Do this workout 3 times a week on non-consecutive days, such as Mon., Wed., and Fri. | Do three sets of 25 to 30 reps. | A pair of 15- to 20-pound (7- to 9-kg) dumbbells, a large exercise ball, and a 3-pound (1.5-kg) ball |
| **WORKOUT 4:**<br>super advanced<br><br>Reverse Single-Leg Lunge on Step<br>Single-Leg Deadlift with Dumbbells<br>Cross-Over Leg Booty Plank<br> on Big Ball | ○○○○ | OhMyGod! Gives you a rock-hard tushy! | 15 to 20 minutes | Do this workout 3 times a week on non-consecutive days, such as Mon., Wed., and Fri. | Do three sets of 25 to 30 reps. | A pair of 10- to 20-pound (4.5- to 9-kg) dumbbells, stability ball, and a step with a set of risers |

○○○○
**WORKOUT 1:**
# beginner

squat with dumbbells
deadlift with dumbbells
booty hydrant

---

**THE PAYOFF:**
## Gets you bootyluscious— and sexy cheeky!

---

**TOTAL TIME:** 15 to 20 minutes

**HOW OFTEN:** Spend two to four weeks building the supporting muscles of your hams and glutes to stay injury-free in the more advanced workouts. Do this workout three times a week on nonconsecutive days.

★ **BOOTY FOCUS,**
on page 100, offers more advice
for maximizing this workout.

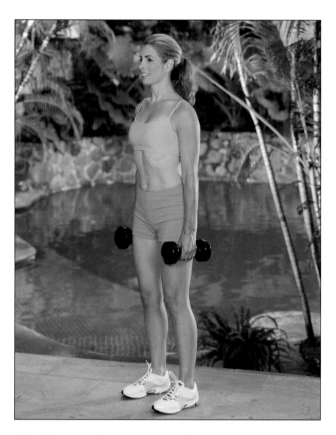

**STARTING POSITION:** Stand with your feet a little wider than hip-width apart and hold a 10- to 15-pound (4.5- to 7-kg) dumbbell in each hand. Look forward and slightly up.

## the payoff:

Burns your buns—in a good way!

# dumbbells

**sets -n- reps:** Do three sets of 15 to 20 reps.
**must-haves:** A pair of 10- to 15-pound (4.5- to 7-kg) dumbbells

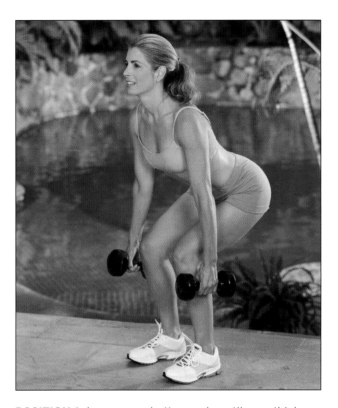

**POSITION 1:** Lower your bottom only until your thighs are parallel to the floor, knees aligned with your second and third toes. Keep your chest lifted and your spine straight, with the majority of your body weight in your heels. Return to starting position. Do 15 to 20 reps.

## FABULOUS FORM TIPS

○ Don't lean forward. Your torso will naturally come forward slightly as you squat. Sit in your heels; imagine that you're sitting in a chair so your heiny leads the way and hold the squat for 2 seconds (count one 1,000, two 2,000) to get maximus backside results.

○ Don't turn your knees in. Keep them stable and point your toes forward as you squat down.

○ Do use sexy posture. Straighten your spine from the top of your head and down, and relax your shoulders.

○ Don't overarch your lower back. Turn on your abs to provide support for your lower back.

# **1** deadlift with dumbbells

○○○○

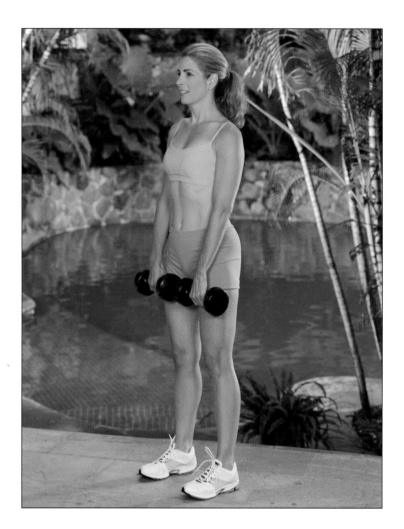

**STARTING POSITION:** Stand hip-width apart, with your knees straight. Hold a 10- to 15-pound (4.5- to 7-kg) dumbbell in each hand.

## the payoff:

Lifts your underbutt!

**sets -n- reps:**  Do three sets of 15 to 20 reps.

**must-haves:**  A pair of 10- to 15-pound (4.5- to 7-kg) dumbbells

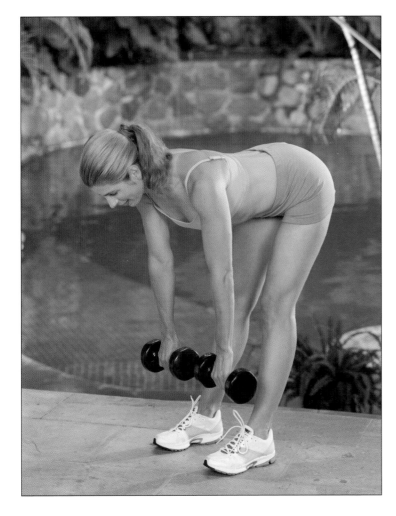

**POSITION 1:** Bend at the waist, chest forward, and keep your legs straight or slightly bend your knees. Lift your navel to your spine to support your lower back as you return to the starting position. Do 15 to 20 reps.

## FABULOUS FORM TIPS

❍ Don't round your spine. Keep your torso straight and your head in line with your spine.

❍ Don't do this exercise if you have a lower back injury. Check with your doctor first.

❍ Don't hang in your lower back; lift your belly button to your spine to engage your abs and support your lower back.

❍ Do engage your underbutt. Truly, this exercise is the best for that prone-to-droop area under your panties!

# **1** booty hydrant

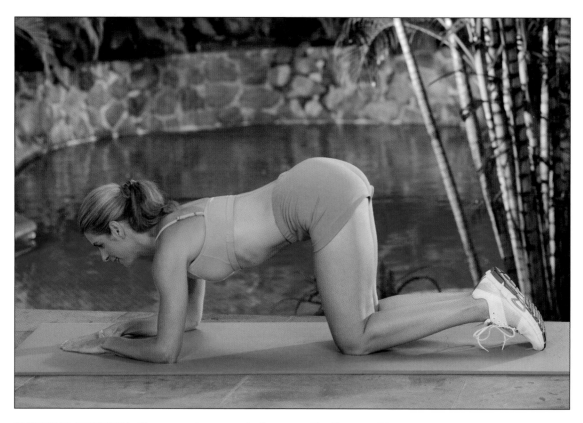

**sets -n- reps:** Do three sets of 15 to 20 reps.
**must-haves:** Nothing

**STARTING POSITION:** Place your knees and elbows on the floor, making sure that your knees are directly under your hipbones. Look down.

## the payoff:

Perks up your bum!

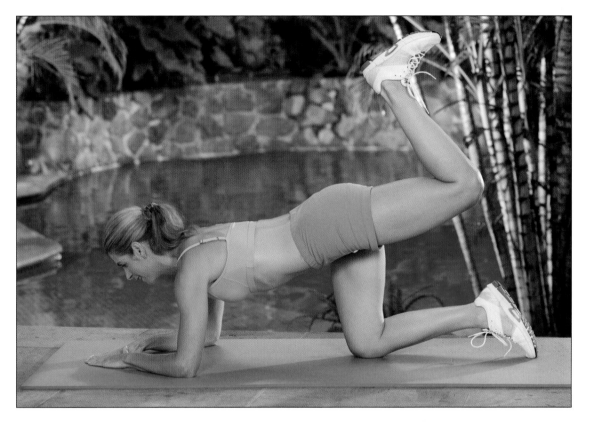

**POSITION 1:** Lift your left leg up, flexing your foot as if making an imprint of your heel on the ceiling. Your knee should be in line with your hipbones. Squeeze your booty and then lift your leg an inch or so to the ceiling. Focus on the contraction as your press your heel toward the ceiling. Do 15 to 20 reps.

## FABULOUS FORM TIPS

❍ Don't lift your knee too high. Instead, fire up your maximus and work it until you feel the burn.

❍ Use your abs to help stabilize your trunk. Lift your belly button to your spine and keep the movement oh-so-small to get major booty benefits.

❍ Don't frantically lift and lower your leg. Use slow and controlled movements to isolate your heiny. It's the only way to de-jiggle your junk!

❍ Turn on your underbutt; imagine putting a pencil under the cheeky droopy area and holding it the whole time.

## ●●○○

### WORKOUT 2:
# intermediate

froggy on big ball
lateral squat with dumbbell
leg lifts on ball

---

**THE PAYOFF:**
## Gives you goddess-worthy, grabbable glutes!

**TOTAL TIME:** 15 to 20 minutes

**HOW OFTEN:** Spend two to four weeks beautifying your booty. Do this workout three times a week on nonconsecutive days.

**★ BOOTY FOCUS,**
**on page 100, offers more advice**
**for maximizing this workout.**

---

# **2** froggy on big ball
○○○○

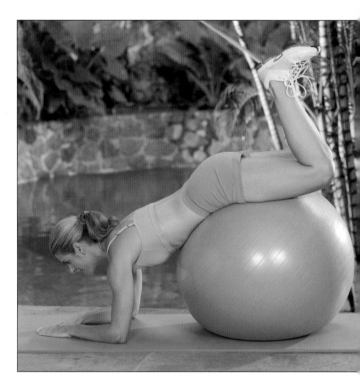

**STARTING POSITION:** Kneel in front of the ball and drape your belly and hips over the ball. Roll on your hips so the ball supports your torso. Place your elbows on the floor in front of the ball and then open your legs slightly to bend your knees, placing your heels together. Gaze at the floor.

## the payoff:
Tones and tightens your gorgeous glutes!

**sets -n- reps:** Do three sets of 15 to 25 reps.

**must-haves:** A large exercise ball. (You can do the exercises on the floor if you don't have a ball.)

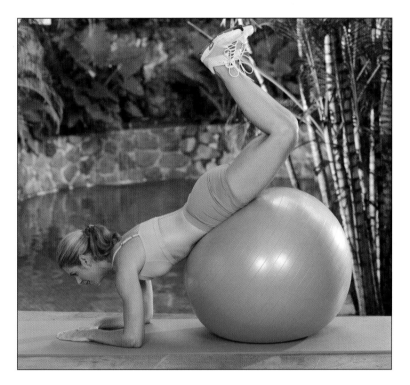

**POSITION 1:** Inhale to lift your feet to the ceiling and then exhale to lower your knees to the ball. If you need rest, drape yourself over the ball after you're done to get a yummy lower back stretch.

## FABULOUS FORM TIPS

❍ Don't pooch your belly. Instead, lift your belly button to your spine the whole time to support your lower back.

❍ Don't forget to firm up your fanny. Imagine holding a $1,000 bill between your butt cheeks.

❍ Firm up your underbutt. Imagine pencils under your butt cheeks to de-droop it, too!

# **2** lateral squat with dumbbell

○○○○

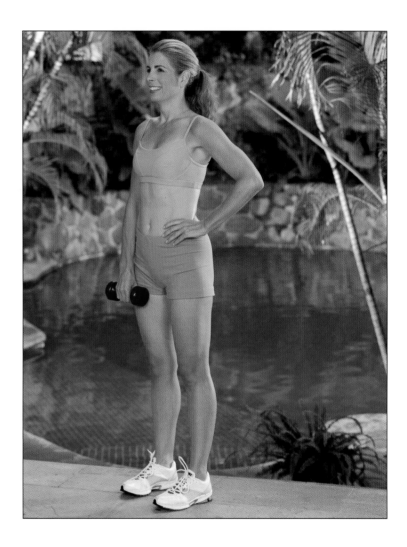

**STARTING POSITION:** Stand with your legs together. Hold an 8- to 10-pound (3.5- to 4.5-kg) dumbbell in your right hand and place your left hand on your hip.

## the payoff:

Sexifies your butt-n-inner thighs

**sets -n- reps:** Do three sets of 15 to 25 reps.

**must-haves:** An 8- to 15-pound (3.5- to 7-kg) dumbbell

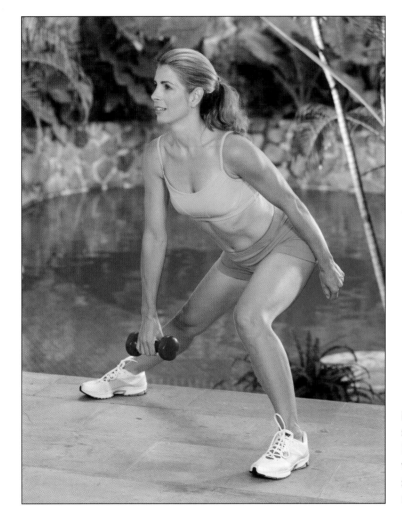

**POSITION 1:** Step to the left and then squat, making sure you put the majority of your body weight in the left leg while the right leg remains completely straight. Do 15 to 25 reps, and then repeat on your right side.

## FABULOUS FORM TIPS

○ Don't lean forward. For your best booty results, the majority of your body weight should be in the heel of your squat leg.

○ Engage your abs to support your lower back and help keep you steady.

○ Don't swing your dumbbell as you move to the side.

○ Squeeze your booty as you push off the squat leg. You're getting inner thigh "bennies," too.

# **2** leg lifts on ball

○○○○

**sets -n- reps:** Do three sets of 15 to 25 reps.

**must-haves:** A large exercise ball. (You can do the exercises on the floor if you don't have a ball.)

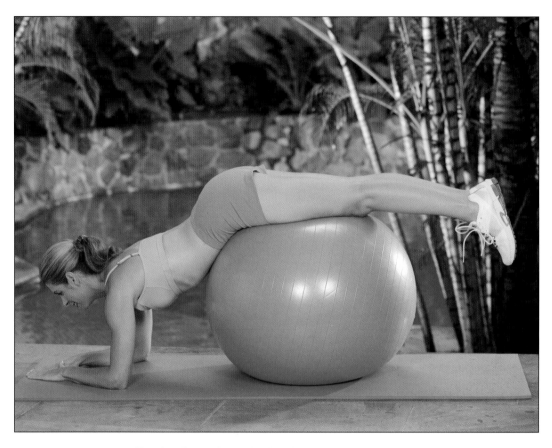

**STARTING POSITION:** Kneel in front of your ball and drape your belly and hips over the ball. Roll on your hips so the ball supports your torso. Place your elbows on the floor in front of the ball. Gaze at the floor. Lift your legs, engaging your glutes, heels together.

## the payoff:

Leaves you cheeky-sexy!

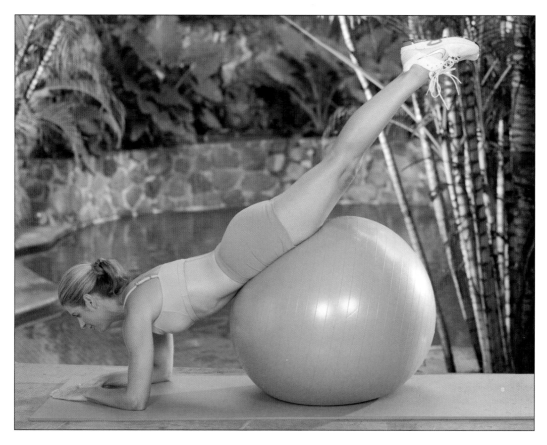

**POSITION 1:** Lift your legs and lower them, lifting from your underbutt. If you need a rest, drape yourself over ball after you're done for a yummy lower back stretch.

## FABULOUS FORM TIPS

○ Don't let your belly sag. Lift your belly button to your spine the whole time to support your lower back. Try exhaling as you lift your legs to support your back.

○ Don't forget to firm up your fanny. Put a pencil between your butt cheeks. Well, at least imagine it!

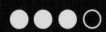

## WORKOUT 3:
# advanced

walking lunges
booty hydrant with
3-pound (1.5-kg) ball
plié squat

---

**THE PAYOFF:**
## Kicks your underbutt!

---

**TOTAL TIME:** 15 to 20 minutes.

**HOW OFTEN:** Now that you're in advanced territory, do this as long as you would like to keep your bum beautiful. But don't forget you need to challenge those muscles three times a week on nonconsecutive days.

★ **BOOTY FOCUS,**
on page 100, offers more advice
for maximizing this workout.

# **3** walking lunges
○○○○

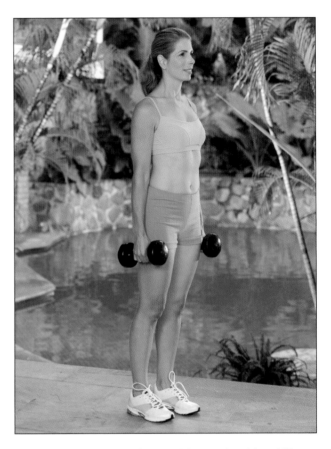

**STARTING POSITION:** Stand with your feet hip-width apart and hold a 15- to 20-pound (7- to 9-kg) dumbbell in each hand.

## the payoff:

Strengthens and slims your underbutt!

**sets -n- reps:** Do three sets of 25 to 30 reps.

**must-haves:** A pair of 15- to 20-pound (7- to 9-kg) dumbbells

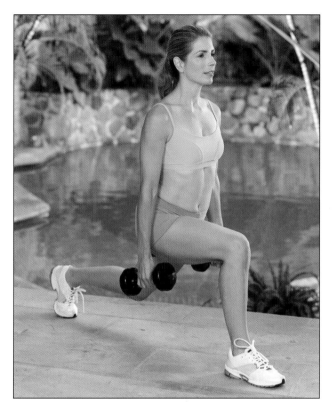 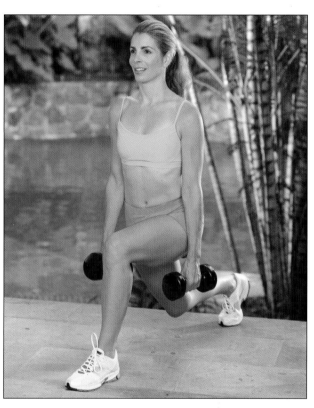

**POSITION 1:** Step forward with your right foot to lower your body in a lunge. Your right thigh should be parallel to the floor while your left thigh is perpendicular to the floor. (Your left knee should aim toward the floor.)

**POSITION 2:** Walk your left foot up to your right foot, come to a standing position, and then lunge forward with the left leg. Keep your spine straight and lifted as you walk. Do 20 reps on each leg.

## FABULOUS FORM TIPS

❍ Don't lean forward. Align your knee over your second and third toes, keeping your body weight in the lunge leg.

❍ Don't round your spine. Instead, keep your chest lifted, shoulders relaxed, and toes pointing forward.

❍ Use your abs to support your lower back.

❍ Hold your lunge for two seconds (count one 1,000, two 2,000) to tackle the toughest of dimples.

# **3** booty hydrant with 3-pound (1.5-kg)

○○○○

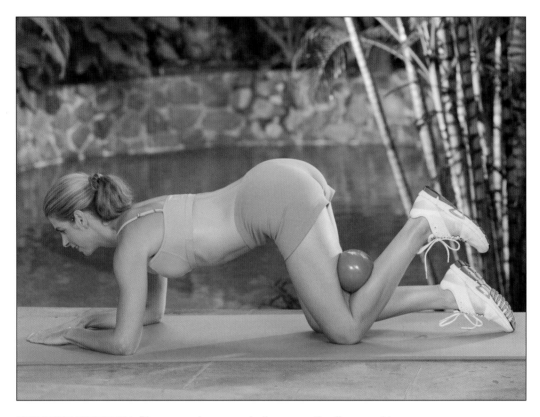

**STARTING POSITION:** Place your knees and elbows on the floor, making sure that your knees are directly under your hipbones. Lift your left knee slightly and place a 3-pound (1.5-kg) ball behind it. Look down.

## **the payoff:**

Tackles the hard to get to area—right underneath your panties!

# ball

**sets -n- reps:** Do three sets of 25 to 30 reps.
**must-haves:** A 3-pound (1.5-kg) ball

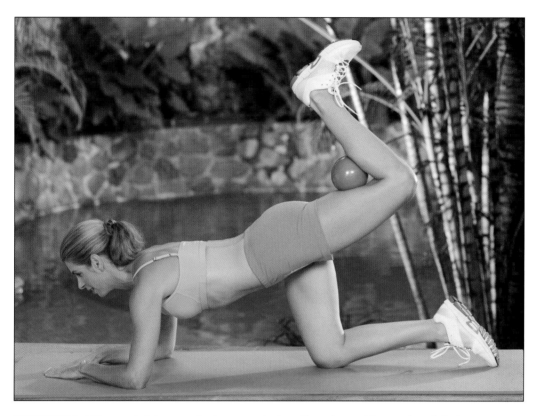

**POSITION 1:** Lift your left leg up, flexing your foot as if you're making an imprint of your heel on the ceiling. Your knee should be in line with your hipbones. Squeeze your booty and then lift your leg only an inch or so to the ceiling. Engage your bum as you press your heel toward the ceiling. Do 25 to 30 reps, then switch legs.

## FABULOUS FORM TIPS

❍ Don't lift your knee too high, otherwise you may feel this in your lower back. The idea is to isolate your booty, girl!

❍ Use your abs to help stabilize your trunk. Lift your belly button to your spine and keep tension on your booty for major booty benefits.

❍ Don't frantically lift and lower your leg; use slow and controlled movements to isolate your heiny. It's the only way to de-jiggle!

❍ Turn on your underbutt; imagine putting a pencil under the cheeky, droopy area, holding it the whole time.

# **3** plié squat

**sets -n- reps:** Do three sets of 25 to 30 reps.
**must-haves:** A 15- to 20-pound (7- to 9-kg) dumbbell

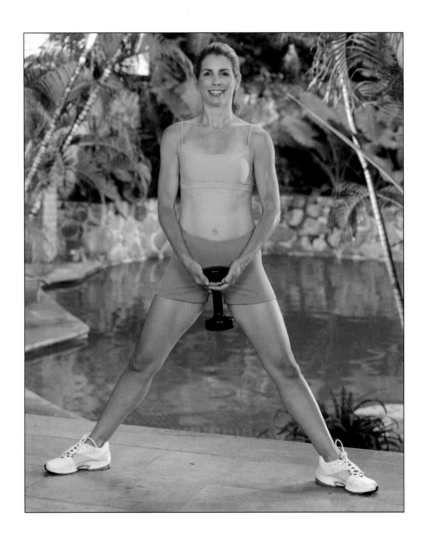

**STARTING POSITION:** Stand with your feet about three feet apart (twice hip-width) and turn out your toes. Hold a 15- to 20-pound (7- to 9-kg) dumbbell in your hands. Look forward and slightly up.

## the payoff:

Thins your "tuckus"— and thighs, too!

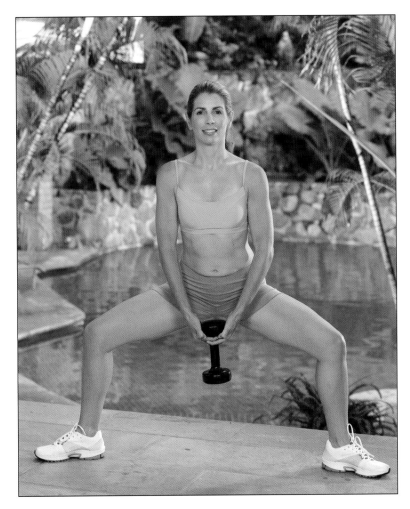

**POSITION 1:** Lower your bottom only until your thighs are parallel to the floor and your knees are aligned with your second and third toes. Keep your chest lifted and your spine straight, with the majority of your body weight in your heels. Do 25 to 30 reps.

## FABULOUS FORM TIPS

○ Don't turn your knees in. Focus on putting the majority of your body weight on the outside edges of your feet.

○ Squeeze your bottom when you lift up—major underbutt benefits!

○ Use sexy posture. Straighten your spine from the top of your head and down and relax your shoulders.

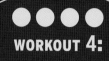

**WORKOUT 4:**

# super advanced

reverse single-leg lunge
(stationary) on step
single-leg deadlift with dumbbells
cross-over leg booty
plank on big ball

---

**THE PAYOFF:**
## OhMyGod! Gives you a rock-hard tushy!

---

**TOTAL TIME:** 15 to 20 minutes

**HOW OFTEN:** Keep it up, cookie! Go with this workout as long as you would like, three times a week on nonconsecutive days.

★ **BOOTY FOCUS,**
on page 100, offers more advice
for maximizing this workout.

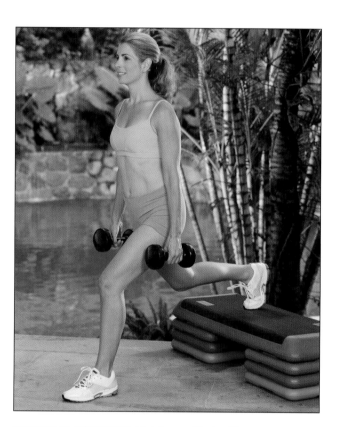

**STARTING POSITION:** Holding a 10- to 20-pound (4.5- to 9-kg) dumbell in each hand, stand in front of your step and turn sideways to place your right foot on the step (about four risers high) or on stairs. Get into a lunge position with your foot on top of the step. Your thigh should be parallel to the step. Your hip points face forward. Engage your abs.

## the payoff:
Transforms a bum from
flabulous to fabulous!

# lunge on step

**sets -n- reps:** Do three sets of 25 to 30 reps.
**must-haves:** A step with a set of risers

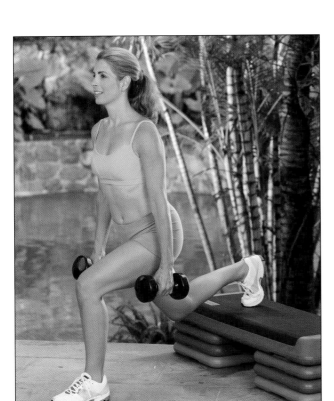

**POSITION 1:** Stabilize in a lunge and then lower and lift, sinking into your hip to work your butt. Lift from the top of your head and drop your shoulders. Do as many as you can with good form, ideally 25 to 30 reps, then switch legs.

## FABULOUS FORM TIPS

○ Don't move your leg on the step. Instead, sink deep into the lunge leg to turn on your maximus.

○ Don't move your knee. Push through your heel to stabilize your lunge leg.

○ Don't round your upper back; sexy posture, pleeease!

# **4** single-leg deadlift with dumbbells

○○○○

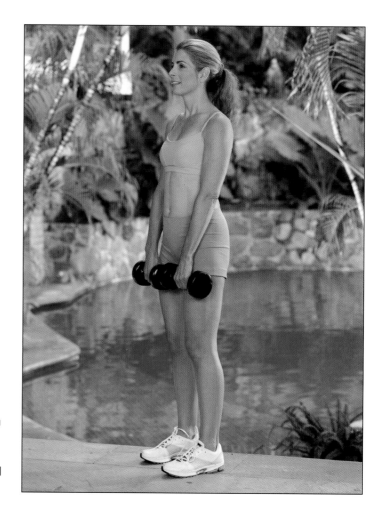

**STARTING POSITION:** Stand with your feet hip-width apart, with your knees straight. Hold a 10- to 20-pound (4.5- to 9-kg) dumbbell in each hand.

## **the payoff:**

Delivers "hanky-panky" results

**sets -n- reps:** Do three sets of 25 to 30 reps.

**must-haves:** A pair of 10- to 20-pound (4.5- to 9-kg) dumbbells

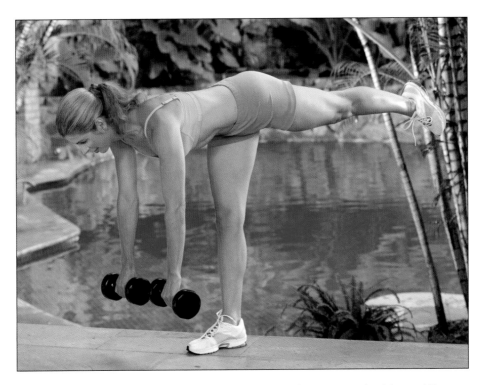

**POSITION 1:** At the same time, bend at your waist, lower your chest toward the floor, and lift your left leg behind you, keeping your head in line with your spine. Lift your navel to the sky, and then lift your torso to a standing position. Do 25 to 30 reps, and then switch legs.

## FABULOUS FORM TIPS

❍ Don't round your spine. Keep your torso straight and your head in line with your spine.

❍ Don't do this exercise if you have a lower back injury. Check with your doctor first.

❍ Don't hang in your lower back. Instead, lift your belly button to your spine to engage your abs and support your lower back.

❍ Engage your underbutt. This exercise is truly the best for that prone-to-droop area under your panties!

# **4** cross-over leg booty plank on big ball

○○○○

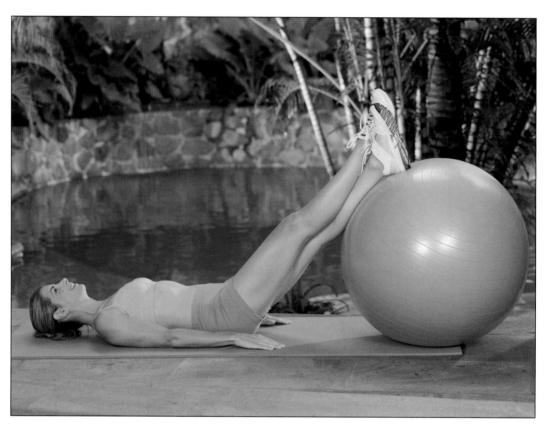

**STARTING POSITION:** Lie on your back with a large ball under your heels. Straighten your arms by your sides, with your palms down. Cross your right leg over your left leg.

## **the payoff:**

Simply "Di" best butt!

**sets -n- reps:** Do three sets of 25 to 30 reps.
**must-haves:** Stability ball

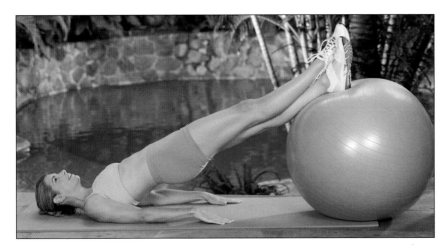

**POSITION 1:** Lift your hips to the sky so your back is off of the floor.

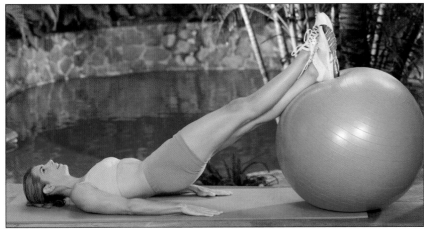

**POSITION 2:** Lower your bum toward the floor, about halfway down, and then squeeze your booty to lift your bum up. Do 25 to 30 reps, and then switch legs.

# FABULOUS FORM TIPS

- Don't drop your hips to the floor. The focus is on the contraction as you lift your hips.

- Stay strong in your core and engage your butt to keep your hips even and your pelvis stable.

- Don't sag anywhere. Your breastbone and pubic bone should form one line as you finish the exercise.

- Use your arms. Press the palms of your hands into the floor to help keep you steady while working your legs.

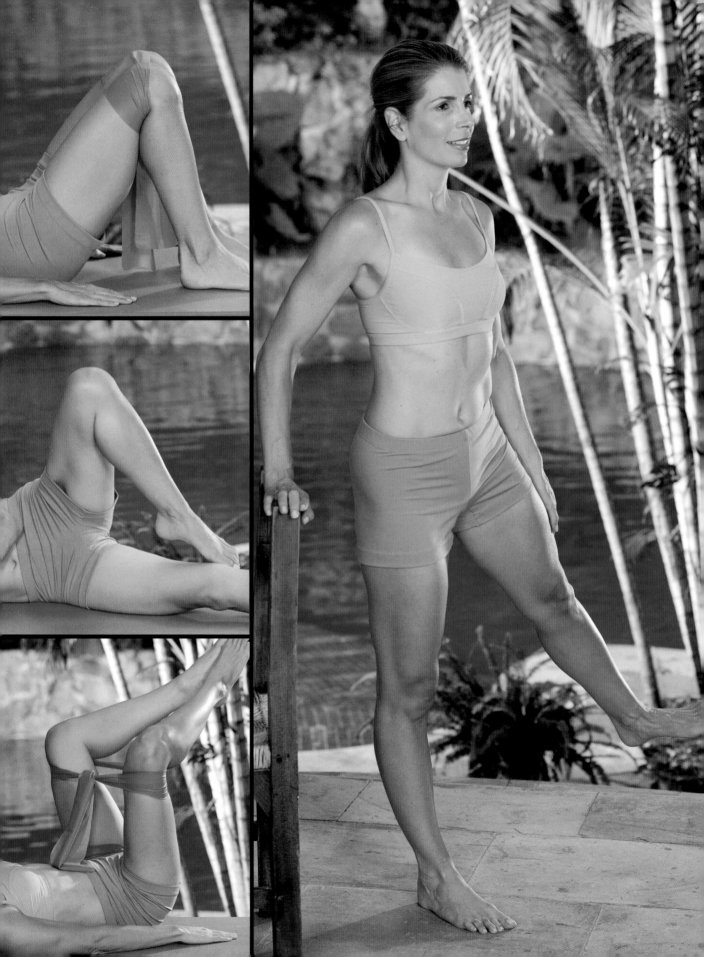

# chapter 5

# SLIMTASTIC OUTER THIGHS

| | the payoff | total time | how often | sets -n- reps | must-haves |
|---|---|---|---|---|---|
| **WORKOUT 1:** ○○○○<br>beginner<br>Clam with Resistance Band<br>Side Passé<br>Bridge with Outer Thigh Press<br>  (Resistance Band) | De-dimples, de-droops, making those thighs de-lovely! | 15 to 20 minutes | Do this workout 3 times a week on non-consecutive days, such as Mon., Wed., and Fri. | Do three sets of 15 to 20 reps. | Light or medium resistance band |
| **WORKOUT 2:** ○○○○<br>intermediate<br>Outer Thigh Lifts with Resistance Band<br>Hot Potato with Resistance Band<br>Hydrant Outer Thigh | Melts the (uninvited) inches! | 15 to 20 minutes | Do this workout 3 times a week on non-consecutive days, such as Mon., Wed., and Fri. | Do three sets of 20 to 25 reps. | Medium resistance band |
| **WORKOUT 3:** ○○○○<br>advanced<br>Standing Outer Thigh Lifts<br>Leg Lift Combo with Resistance Band<br>Clam with Resistance Band<br>  (on Your Back) | Super-slenders all of the saddlebag places! | 15 to 20 minutes | Do this workout 3 times a week on non-consecutive days, such as Mon., Wed., and Fri. | Do three sets of 25 to 30 reps. | Medium resistance band |
| **WORKOUT 4:** ○○○○<br>super advanced<br>Outer Thigh Lifts with Ankle Weights<br>Hot Potato Plus with Ankle Weights<br>Standing Outer Thigh Lifts<br>  with Ankle Weights | Gets your legs backyard, bikini, or beach ready! | 15 to 20 minutes | Do this workout 3 times a week on non-consecutive days, such as Mon., Wed., and Fri. | Do three sets of 25 to 30 reps. | Pair of 5-pound (2-kg) ankle weights or a medium resistance band |

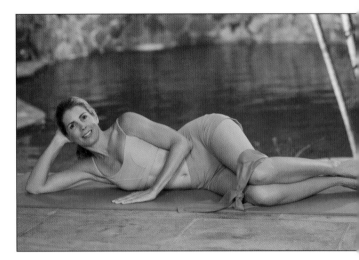

**STARTING POSITION:** Tie a band tightly around your thighs, near your knees. Lie on your right side with your knees bent and place them in front of your torso so your ankles, knees, and hipbones are stacked. Prop your head up with your right arm and then place your left arm, palm down, on the mat in front of your torso; relax your shoulders.

●○○○

## WORKOUT 1:
# beginner

clam with resistance band
side passé
bridge with outer thigh press
(resistance band)

---

### THE PAYOFF:
## De-dimples, de-droops, making those thighs de-lovely!

---

**TOTAL TIME:** 15 to 20 minutes

**HOW OFTEN:** Spend two to four weeks to learn how to hold your body correctly and build strength for more advanced work to come. Don't rush ahead too soon. Breathe normally. Do this workout three times a week on nonconsecutive days.

★ **RESIZE YOUR THIGHS,** on page 100, offers more advice for maximizing this workout.

## the payoff:
Thighs that'll turn eyes!

# resistance band

**sets -n- reps:** Do three sets of 15 to 20 reps or more.

**must-haves:** Light or medium resistance band

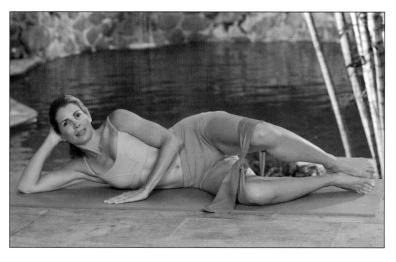

**POSITION 1:** Lift your top leg toward the ceiling, keeping your knees stacked. Lower your leg. Do 15 to 20 reps.

## FABULOUS FORM TIPS

❍ Don't lift too high. You should feel this work in the outer thigh. If you lift too high, you may feel strain higher on your hip (such as underneath the hipbone) and thus miss out on the juicy outer thigh work. Think saddlebag area.

❍ Focus on keeping your knees together.

❍ Focus and squeeze your outer thigh as you lift your leg to isolate the outer thigh muscles and super-tone your legs.

❍ If the resistance band is too hard, then just do the exercise without the band.

# 1 side passé

○○○○

| | |
|---|---|
| **sets -n- reps:** | Do three sets of 15 to 20 reps or more. |
| **must-haves:** | Nothing |

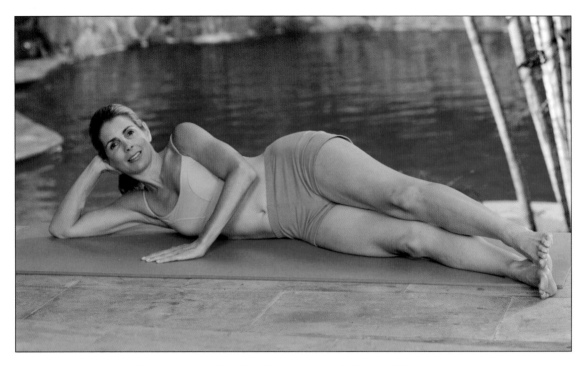

**STARTING POSITION:** Lie on your right side with your legs straight, ankles, knees, and hipbones stacked on top of one another. Prop your head up with your right arm and then place your left arm, palm down, on the mat in front of your torso. Relax your shoulders. Lift both legs at the same time and lower them in front of your body to about a 45-degree angle so your body makes the shape of a banana.

## the payoff:

Whittles away wide thighs!

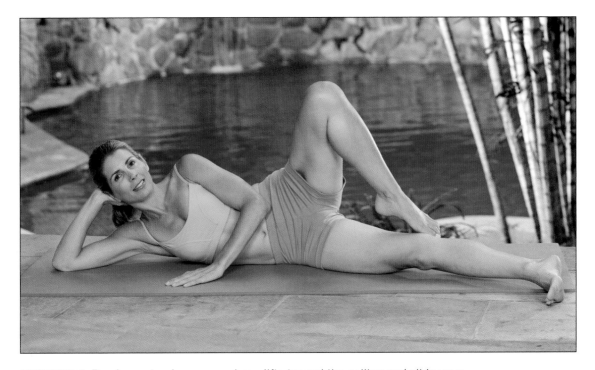

**POSITION 1:** Bend your top leg so your knee lifts toward the ceiling and slide your toes along the inside of your bottom leg. Then straighten your legs, sliding your toes along the inside of your thighs (back to the starting position). This gives you more thigh action. Do 15 to 20 reps.

## FABULOUS FORM TIPS

○ Don't sit back in your hips. If your hips are tight, it may be hard to open your leg so your knee lifts to the ceiling, causing you to sit back. Focus on squeezing your outer thighs before lifting your knee to the ceiling to open your hips.

○ Squeeze your thighs when you're moving your leg back and forth.

○ Lift your knee to the ceiling (so you can isolate your outer thigh) during the entire exercise.

# **1** bridge with outer thigh press

○○○○

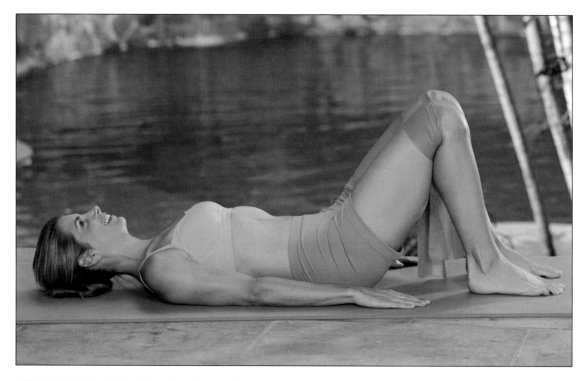

**STARTING POSITION:** Tie a band around your legs, just above your knees, and then lie on your back with your knees bent and straighten your arms by your sides.

## the payoff:

Erases your bumps on your bum and on your thighs!
Whoohoo!

# (resistance band)

**sets -n- reps:** Do three sets of 15 to 20 reps or more.
**must-haves:** Light or medium resistance band

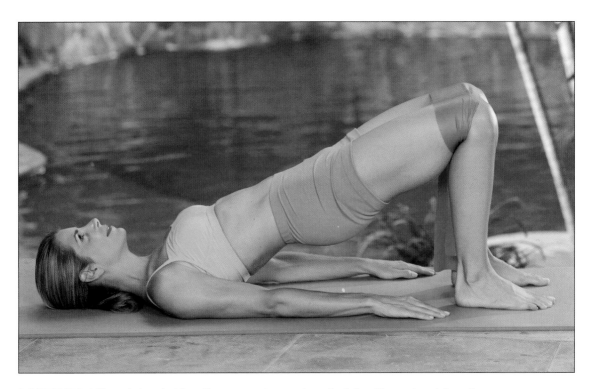

**POSITION 1:** Lift up into a bridge. Press your legs out against the fitness band, keeping resistance on the band the whole time; squeeze and release. Do 15 to 20 reps.

## FABULOUS FORM TIPS

○ Align your feet under your knees and walk your feet back until you can almost touch them with your hands.

○ Push out from your outer thighs to get the ultra-delicious outer thigh work.

●●○○

**WORKOUT 2:**
# intermediate

outer thigh lifts
with resistance band
hot potato
with resistance band
hydrant outer thigh

---

**THE PAYOFF:**
## Melts the (uninvited) inches!

---

**TOTAL TIME:** 15 to 20 minutes

**HOW OFTEN:** Now the focus is engaging to isolate your outer thigh muscles, which are hidden under those saddlebags. So really squeeze before moving! First do all of the exercises lying on your right side. After you complete the Hydrant Outer Thigh, switch legs and repeat the sequence lying on your left side. Breathe normally. Do this workout three times a week on nonconsecutive days.

★ **RESIZE YOUR THIGHS,**
on page 100, offers more advice
for maximizing this workout.

# 2  outer thigh lifts
○○○○

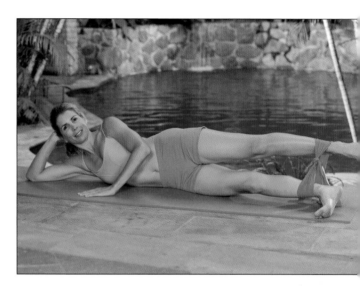

**STARTING POSITION:** Tie a band around your ankles. (Tie it pretty tightly, but you want to be able to move your leg behind you, so experiment.) Lie on your right side with your legs straight, and your ankles, knees, and hip-bones stacked on top of one another. Prop your head up with your right arm and then place your left arm, palm down, on the mat in front of your torso; relax your shoulders. Lift both legs at the same time and lower them in front of your body to about a 45-degree angle. Move your top leg behind you, so that your toes are parallel.

## the payoff:
Sculpts shapely legs!

# with resistance band

**sets -n- reps:** Do three sets of 20 to 25 reps.
**must-haves:** Medium resistance band

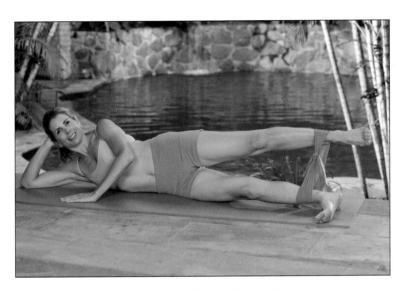

**POSITION 1:** Lift your top leg to hip height, and then lower, keeping the tension on the fitness band the whole time. Do 20 to 25 reps.

## FABULOUS FORM TIPS

○ Don't move your hips. They should remain stacked and stable as you lower and lift your leg.

○ Don't lift too high because you may feel this work in your lower back; focus on your outer thigh.

○ Use your abs so you don't feel this in your lower back.

○ Keep tension on the band the whole time. If you feel this in your knees or hips, tie the band around your knees, or don't use the band.

# **2** hot potato with resistance band

○○○○

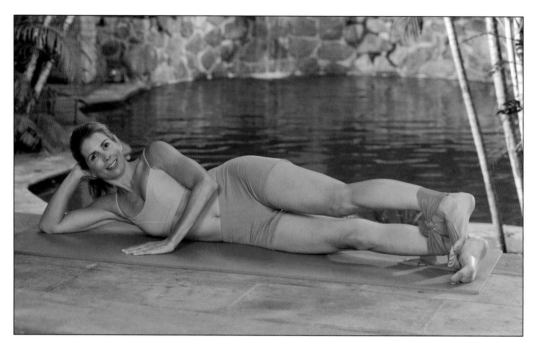

**STARTING POSITION:** Tie a band around your ankles. Lie on your right side with your legs straight, ankles, knees, and hipbones stacked on top of one another. Prop your head up with your right arm and then place your left arm, palm down, on the mat in front of your torso; relax your shoulders. Lift both legs at the same time and lower them in front of your body to about a 45-degree angle. Lift the top leg and turn your toes under as they touch the floor.

## **the payoff:**

Lower and lift for clean legs!

**sets -n- reps:**  Do three sets of 20 to 25 reps.

**must-haves:**  Medium resistance band

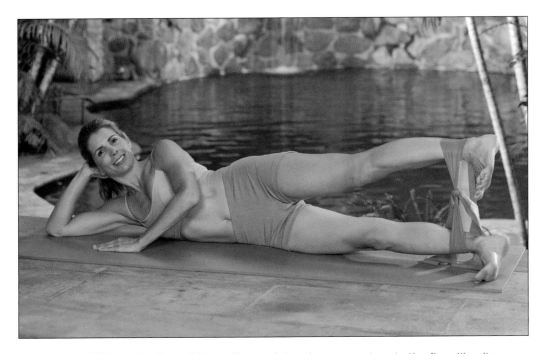

**POSITION 1:** Lift your leg toward the ceiling and then lower your toes to the floor like dipping them in hot water. Dip your toes so they touch the floor. Do 20 to 25 reps.

## FABULOUS FORM TIPS

- Don't move your hips; keep them stacked, using your abs.

- Focus on keeping your toes down so you get lotsa yummy work for the entire thigh!

- Keep the tension on your band the whole time. If you feel this in your lower back, ditch the band and follow the directions without it.

# **2** hydrant outer thigh

○○○○

**sets -n- reps:** Do three sets of 20 to 25 reps.
**must-haves:** Nothing

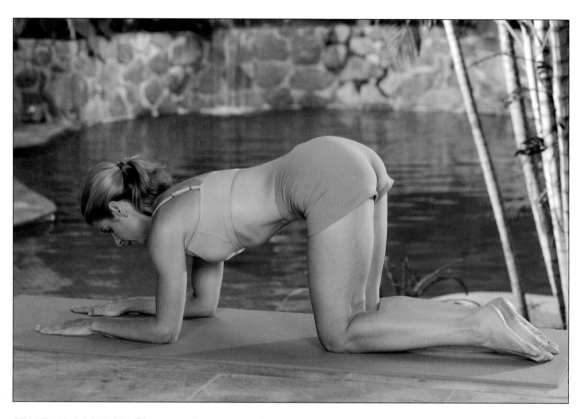

**STARTING POSITION:** Place your knees and elbows on the floor, making sure that your knees are directly under your hipbones. Look down.

## **the payoff:**

Burns lotsa inches!

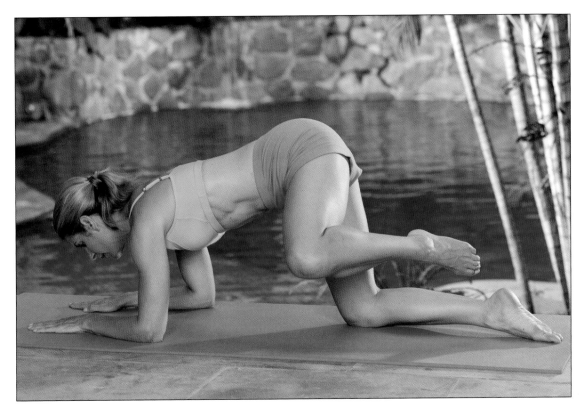

**POSITION 1:** Squeeze your outer thigh, and then lift your left leg up and to the side. Do 20 to 25 reps.

## FABULOUS FORM TIPS

○ Don't lift your leg too high; otherwise, you may feel this in your lower back. The idea is to isolate your outer thigh and work to the point of fatigue.

○ Don't frantically lift and lower your leg. Use slow and controlled movements to isolate those dimples. Say your goodbyes!

○ Don't shift your body to the opposite leg as you lift the working leg. Keep your hips even to keep the tension on the outer thigh of the working leg.

○ Use your abs to help stabilize your trunk and support your lower back. Lift your belly button to your spine the whole time.

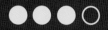
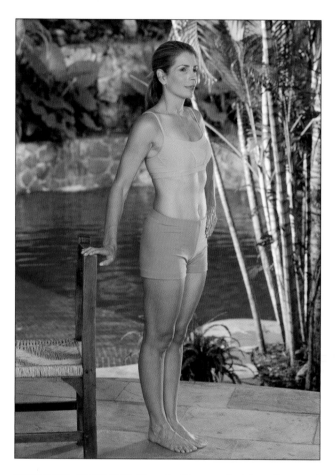

● ● ● ○

**WORKOUT 3:**
# advanced

standing outer thigh lifts

leg lift combo with
resistance band

clam with resistance band
(on your back)

**THE PAYOFF:**
## Super-slenders all of the saddlebag places!

**TOTAL TIME:** 15 to 20 minutes.

**HOW OFTEN:** At this level, you're looking to get rid of the lumps. Stay true to your form, and you'll see the dimples disappear! Start on your left side, and do all the exercises. After Clam on Your Back, repeat the entire sequence on your right side. Breathe normally. Do this workout three days a week on nonconsecutive days.

★ **RESIZE YOUR THIGHS,**
on page 100, offers more advice
for maximizing this workout.

**STARTING POSITION:** Stand with your feet together and parallel and straighten your arms by your sides. Your hipbones should face forward and remain even. Lift from the top of your head and drop your shoulders.

## the payoff:
Smooth, sexy legs!

# thigh lifts

**sets -n- reps:** Do three sets of 25 to 30 reps.
**must-haves:** Nothing

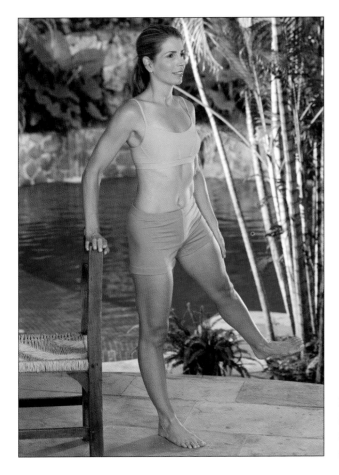

**POSITION 1:** Inhale to lift one leg to the side; keep your foot absolutely parallel to the floor and then exhale to squeeze your inner thighs and slowly lower your leg.

## FABULOUS FORM TIPS

❍ Lift from your hip.

❍ Keep your toes parallel with the floor to isolate your outer thighs.

# **3** leg lift combo with resistance band

○○○○

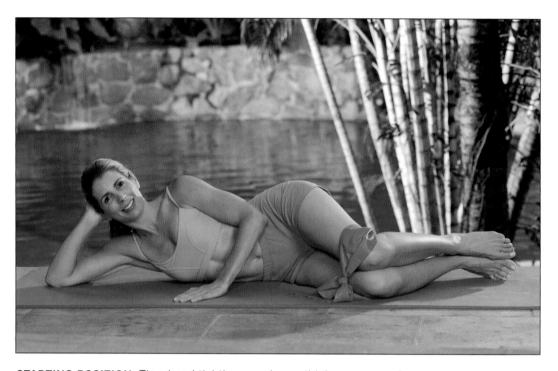

**STARTING POSITION:** Tie a band tightly around your thighs, near your knees, and then lie on your right side with your knees bent and place them in front of your torso so your ankles, knees, and hipbones are stacked. Prop your head up with your right arm and then place your left arm, palm down, on the mat in front of your torso; relax your shoulders.

## **the payoff:**

Seriously wipes out the dimples!

**sets -n- reps:** Do three sets of 25 to 30 reps.

**must-haves:** Medium resistance band

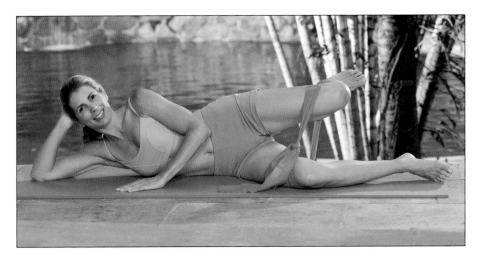

**POSITION 1:** Lift your left leg to hip height and move from front to back so your leg ends up behind your body, flexing your foot. Feel your booty working.

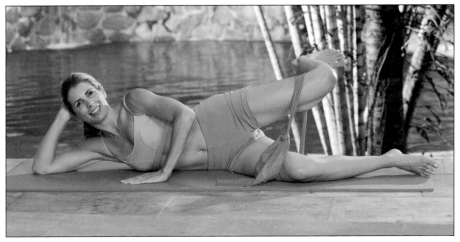

**POSITION 2:** Now, keep your leg behind your body and then lift your leg so you can turn on major thigh work! Do 25 to 30 reps.

# FABULOUS FORM TIPS

○ Don't lift too high; you should feel this work in the outer thigh. If you lift too high, you may miss out on the juicy outer thigh work or stress your hip joints.

○ Focus and squeeze your outer thigh as you lift your leg to feel the oh-so-yummy de-dimple work!

○ Stack your hips to isolate the work. For bonus work, add a combo—bring your leg back (position 1) and then lift up (position 2)—major tushy work!

# **3** clam with resistance band (on your

○○○○

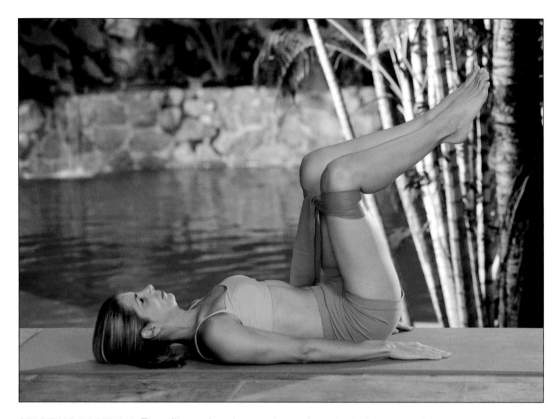

**STARTING POSITION:** Tie a fitness band around your legs, just above your knees, and then lie on your back with your knees bent at a 90-degree angle. Straighten your arms by your sides.

## the payoff:

Delivers OhSo beautiful thighs!

# back)

**sets -n- reps:** Do three sets of 25 to 30 reps.
**must-haves:** Medium resistance band

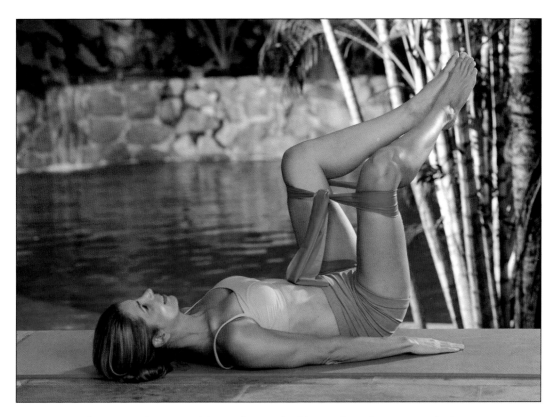

**POSITION 1:** Open your knees, making a diamond with your legs, to press against the fitness band, keeping resistance on the band the whole time; squeeze and release. Do 15 to 20 reps.

## FABULOUS FORM TIPS

❍ Push out from your outer thighs to get the ultra-delicious outer thigh work.

❍ Keep the tension on the band the whole time.

●●●●

**WORKOUT 4:**

# super advanced

outer thigh lifts with ankle weights
hot potato plus with ankle weights
standing outer thigh lifts
with ankle weights

---

**THE PAYOFF:**
## Gets your legs backyard, bikini, or beach ready

---

**TOTAL TIME:** 15 to 20 minutes

**HOW OFTEN:** Keep your movements oh-so-small and controlled. You should feel a little warmth in your outer thigh! You'll use 5-pound (2-kg) ankle weights, but if you're not ready, or if you're traveling, use a light or medium resistance band. Breathe normally. Do this workout three times a week on nonconsecutive days.

★ **RESIZE YOUR THIGHS,**
on page 100, offers more advice for maximizing this workout.

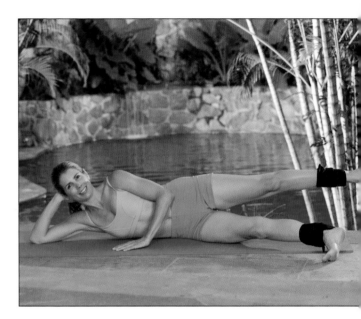

**STARTING POSITION:** Wrap a 5-pound (2-kg) ankle weight around each ankle. Lie on your right side with your legs straight, ankles, knees, and hipbones stacked on top of one another. Prop your head up with your right arm and then place your left arm, palm down, on the mat in front of your torso; relax your shoulders. Lift both legs at the same time and lower them in front of your body to about a 45-degree angle and then move your top leg behind you, toes parallel.

## the payoff:
Delivers OhSo beautiful thighs!

# with ankle weights

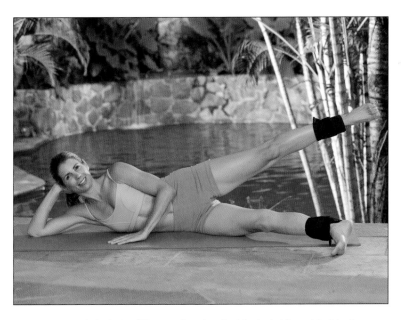

**POSITION 1:** Inhale to lift your top leg to hip height and behind you so it's parallel to the floor, and then exhale to lower your leg to the floor. Do 25 to 30 reps.

## FABULOUS FORM TIPS

- Don't move your hips. They should remain stacked and stable as you lower and lift your leg.

- Don't lift too high. Your goal is to fireup your outer thigh.

- Use your abs to keep your hips stable.

- Work slowly. If you feel this work in your knees or hips, you may not be ready for the added weight. Try it without the ankle weight first.

# **4** hot potato plus with ankle weights

○○○○

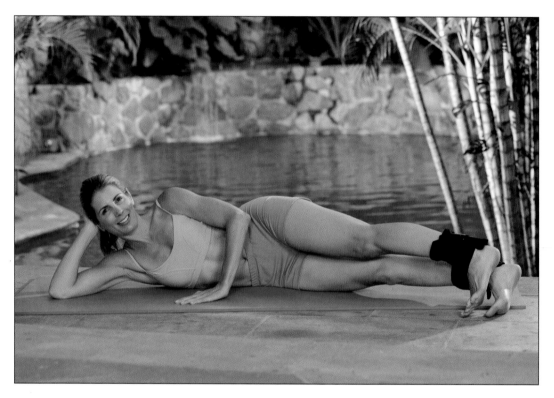

**STARTING POSITION:** Wrap a 5-pound (2-kg) ankle weight around each ankle. Lie on your right side with your legs straight, ankles, knees, and hipbones stacked on top of one another. Prop your head up with your right arm and then place your left arm, palm down, on the mat in front of your torso; relax your shoulders. Lift both legs at the same time and lower them in front of your body to about a 45-degree angle. Lift the top leg and turn your toes under so they are even with your bottom foot.

## **the payoff:**

Gets your legs bikini ready (seriously)!

**sets -n- reps:** Do three sets of whatever it takes, but shoot for 25 to 30 reps!

**must-haves:** 5-pound (2-kg) ankle weights or a medium resistance band

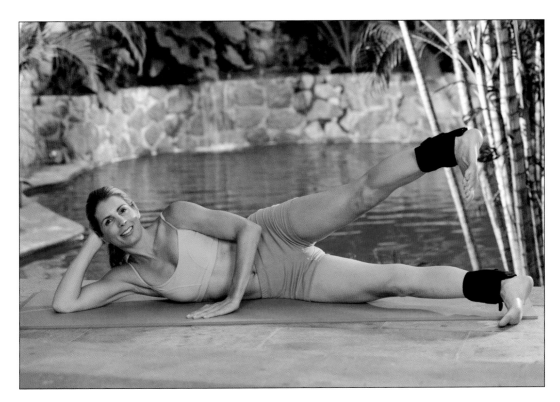

**POSITION 1:** Lift your top leg toward the ceiling as high as you can. (It's tough.) Do 25 to 30 reps.

## FABULOUS FORM TIPS

○ Don't move your hips. Keep them stacked, using your abs.

○ Focus on keeping your toes down so you get lotsa yummy work for the entire thigh!

○ Keep your movements small.

# **4** standing outer thigh lifts with ankle

○○○○

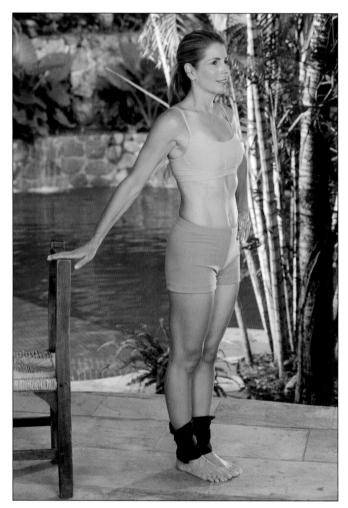

**STARTING POSITION:** Wrap a 5-pound (2-kg) ankle weight around each ankle. Stand with your feet together, parallel with each other, and straighten your arms by your sides. Your hip points should face forward and remain even. Lift from the top of your head and drop your shoulders. Place your fingers on the back of a chair or a wall for support.

## the payoff:

Gets your legs beach ready (of course)!

# weights

**sets -n- reps:** Do three sets of whatever it takes but shoot for 25 to 30 reps!

**must-haves:** 5-pound (2-kg) ankle weights or a medium resistance band

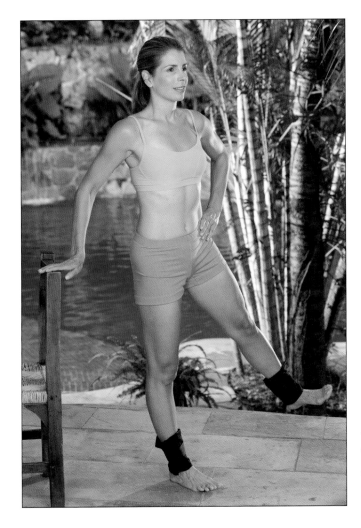

**POSITION 1:** Lift your left leg to the side, not too high, keeping your foot absolutely parallel with the ground, and then slowly lower your leg. Do as many as you can, at least 25 to 30 reps.

## FABULOUS FORM TIPS

○ Lift from your hip.

○ Keep your toes parallel to work your thighs.

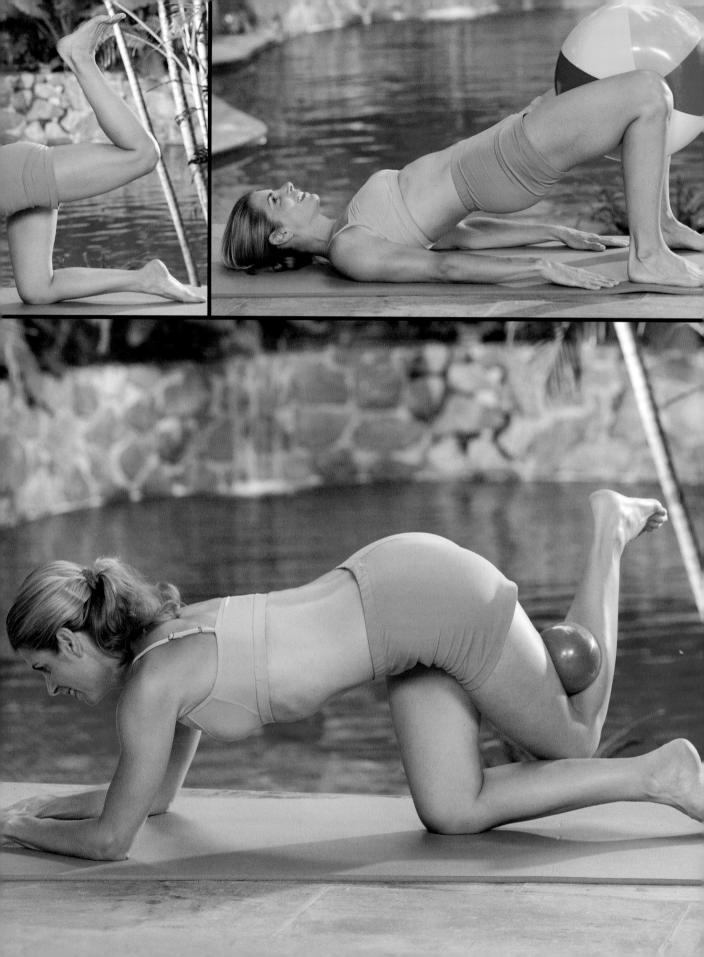

# chapter 6

# SLIMTASTIC INNER THIGHS

| | the payoff | total time | how often | sets -n- reps | must-haves |
|---|---|---|---|---|---|
| **WORKOUT 1:**<br>beginner<br>Inner Thigh Lifts<br>Hydrant Inner Thigh<br>Bridge with Ball Squeeze<br>○○○○ | Strengthens and slims your inner thighs | 15 to 20 minutes | Do this workout 3 times a week on non-consecutive days, such as Mon., Wed., and Fri. | Do three sets of 15 to 20 reps. | Stability ball |
| **WORKOUT 2:**<br>intermediate<br>V Squeeze<br>Hydrant Inner Thigh (Straight Legs)<br>Standing Adduction Leg Lifts<br>○○○○ | Gives you sassy-strong inner thighs! | 15 to 20 minutes | Do this workout 3 times a week on non-consecutive days, such as Mon., Wed., and Fri. | Do three sets of 20 to 25 reps. | Nada |
| **WORKOUT 3:**<br>advanced<br>Inner Thigh Circles with Ankle Weights<br>Hydrant Inner Thigh with 3-pound (1.5-kg) Ball<br>Scissor Legs with Leg Weights<br>○○○○ | Slenderizes your inner thighs! | 15 to 20 minutes | Do this workout 3 times a week on non-consecutive days, such as Mon., Wed., and Fri. | Do three sets of 25 to 30 reps. | 3-pound (1.5-kg) ball and pair of 5-pound (2-kg) ankle weights |
| **WORKOUT 4:**<br>super advanced<br>V Squeeze with Ball<br>Big Ball Beats<br>Standing Adduction Leg Lifts with Ankle Weights<br>○○○○ | Melts your inner thigh flab! | 15 to 20 minutes | Do this workout 3 times a week on non-consecutive days, such as Mon., Wed., and Fri. | Do three sets of 25 to 30 reps. | Stability ball and pair of 5-pound (2-kg) ankle weights |

## WORKOUT 1:
# beginner

inner thigh lifts
hydrant inner thigh
bridge with ball squeeze

---

**THE PAYOFF:**
## Strengthens and slims your inner thighs!

---

**TOTAL TIME:** 15 to 20 minutes

**HOW OFTEN:** Spend two to four weeks to practice good inner thigh transformation. If you need a rest, take it. Breathe normally, unless otherwise indicated. Do this workout three times a week on nonconsecutive days.

★ **RESIZE YOUR THIGHS,**
on page 100, offers more advice
for maximizing this workout.

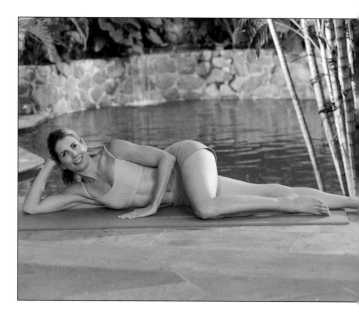

**STARTING POSITION:** Lie on your right side with your left leg bent over your right. Bend your elbow and place your hand under your head for support.

## the payoff:
Simply, thigh-sculpting magic!

**sets -n- reps:** Do three sets of 15 to 20 reps.
**must-haves:** Nothing

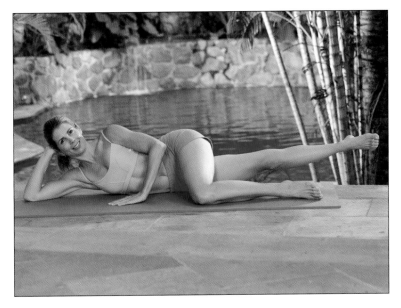

**POSITION 1:** Lift your bottom leg, squeeze your inner thighs, and then lower your leg down. Do 20 to 25 reps.

## FABULOUS FORM TIPS

○ Actively engage your inner thigh from your knee to your groin as you lift your leg. Imagine a bobby pin and how tight it holds together.

○ Don't let your belly sag. Hold it firm so you can isolate those sexy inner thighs.

# 1 hydrant inner thigh

○○○○

**sets -n- reps:** Do three sets of 15 to 20 reps.
**must-haves:** Nothing

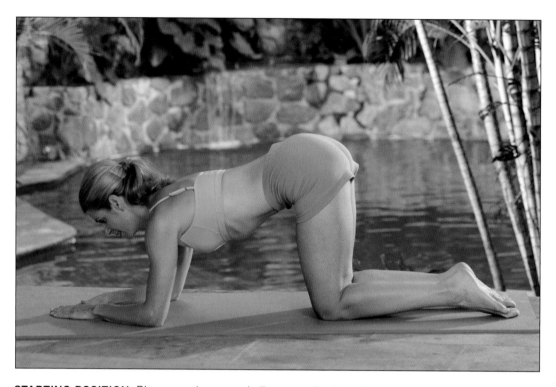

**STARTING POSITION:** Place your knees and elbows on the floor. Relax your head, neck, and shoulders and look down.

## the payoff:

Gets those inner thighs super good-n-skinny

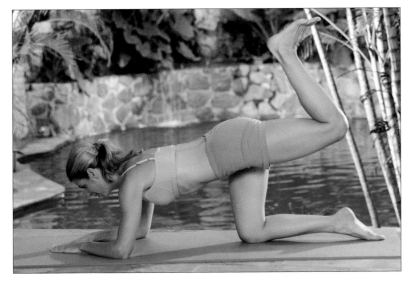

**POSITION 1:** Lift your left leg straight up, leading with your heel as if you're making an imprint of your foot on the ceiling. Squeeze your booty as you lift your leg so your knee is in line with your hip bones.

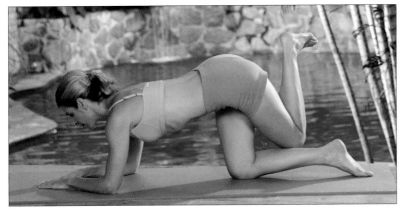

**POSITION 2:** As you lower your leg, cross your knee over your right leg, squeezing your inner thighs scary-tight until you literally feel the contraction between your thighs. Do 15 to 20 reps.

## FABULOUS FORM TIPS

○ Don't forget that the focus is on lowering your leg and squeezing your inner thighs as hard as you can.

○ Don't lift your knee too high; otherwise, you may feel strain in your lower back.

○ Use your booty to get some extra rear work, pushing to the point of a full-on contraction.

○ Use your abs to help stabilize your belly. Lift your belly button to your spine the whole time.

○ Use oh-so-small controlled movements to isolate your inner thighs.

# 1 bridge with ball squeeze

○○○○

**sets -n- reps:** Do three sets of 15 to 20 reps.

**must-haves:** Stability ball. (If you don't have a stability ball, a beach ball will do, anything 15 inches (38 cm) in diameter.)

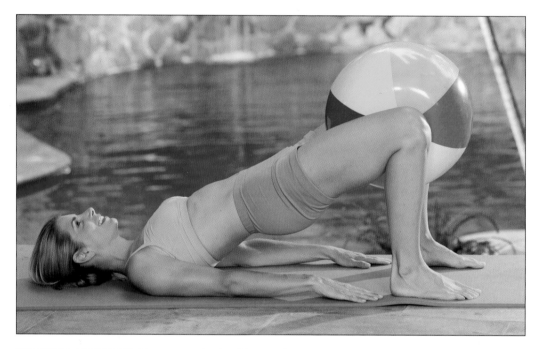

**STARTING POSITION:** Lie on your back with your knees bent at a 90-degree angle and straighten your arms by your sides. Lift up into a bridge. Place a stability or beach ball between your legs and squeeze and release. Do 15 to 20 reps.

## the payoff:

Squeeze for gorgeous inner thighs.

## FABULOUS FORM TIPS

❍ Align your feet under your knees, and walk your feet back until you can almost touch 'em with your hands.

❍ Don't forget to push in to get the ultra-delicious inner thigh work you want.

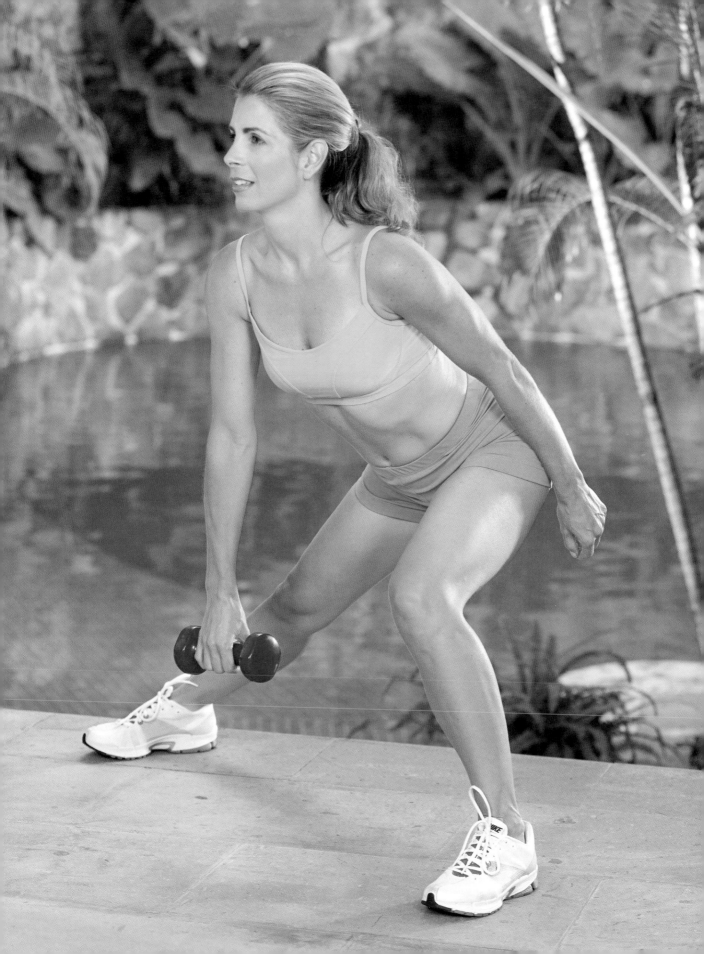

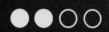

## WORKOUT 2:
# intermediate

v squeeze
hydrant inner thigh (straight legs)
standing adduction leg lifts

**THE PAYOFF:**
Gives you sassy-strong
inner thighs!

**TOTAL TIME:** 15 to 20 minutes

**HOW OFTEN:** Spend two to four weeks really
feeling this work in your inner thighs—engaging
from your knee all the way up to your groin.
Take a break if you need it. Breathe normally.
Do this workout three times a week on
nonconsecutive days.

★ **RESIZE YOUR THIGHS,**
on page 100, offers more advice
for maximizing this workout.

# 2  v squeeze
○○○○

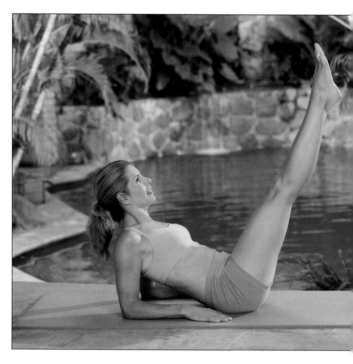

**STARTING POSITION:** Lie back on your elbows, with
your palms down, legs straight in the air.

## the payoff:
Flab-free inner thighs

**sets -n- reps:** Do three sets of 20 to 25 reps.
**must-haves:** Nada

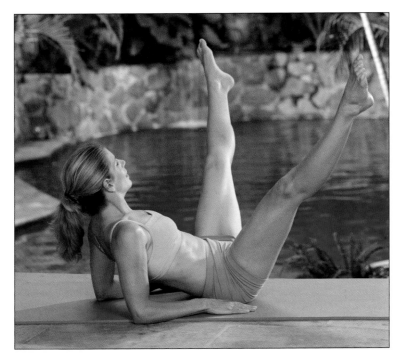

**POSITION 1:** Open your legs to form a V, and then close them slowly, squeezing your inner thighs. Do 20 to 25 reps.

## FABULOUS FORM TIPS

○ Don't forget to fire up your inner thighs, focusing on squeezing them. Remember the bobby pin image.

○ Don't bulge your belly; keep it active to isolate your inner thighs.

○ Keep your legs straight. If you can't straighten your legs because of hamstring tightness, do the same exercise with your knees slightly bent.

# **2** hydrant inner thigh (straight legs)

○○○○

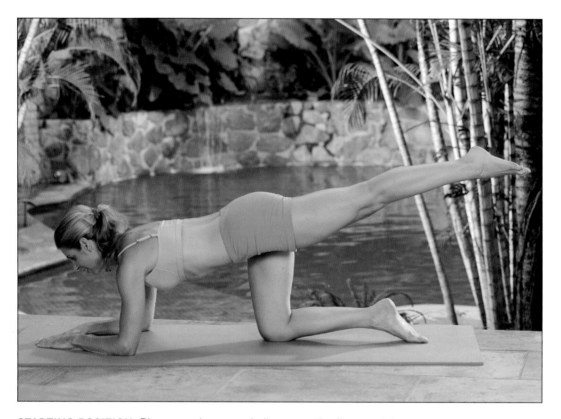

**STARTING POSITION:** Place your knees and elbows on the floor and then straighten your left leg. Relax your head, neck, and shoulders and look down.

## the payoff:

Thins your inner thighs!

**sets -n- reps:**  Do three sets of 20 to 25 reps.
**must-haves:**  Nada

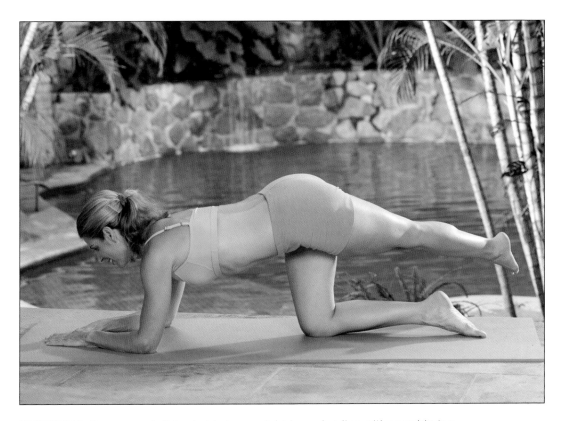

**POSITION 1:** Cross your left leg behind your right knee, leading with your big toe, until you feel the ultra-squeeze in your inner thighs. Never release the contraction as you lower and lift in micro-movements. Do 20 to 25 reps.

## FABULOUS FORM TIPS

○  Don't forget that the focus is on your inner thighs. *Remember the bobby pin image.*

○  Don't lift your leg too high; otherwise, you may feel this work in your lower back.

○  Don't lower and lift your leg frantically. Slow and controlled movements isolate your inner thighs to slenderize 'em!

○  Use your abs to keep your hips stable; lift your belly button to your spine the whole time.

○  Turn on your booty for extra b-side benefits.

# **2** standing adduction leg lifts

○○○○

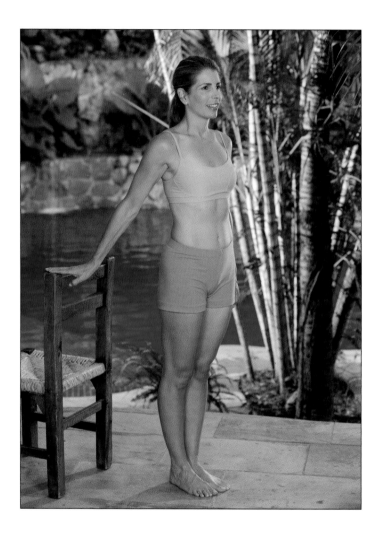

**STARTING POSITION:** Stand with your feet together, parallel with each other, and straighten your arms by your sides. Your hipbones should face forward and remain even. Lift from the top of your head and drop your shoulders. Place your fingertips on a wall or hold the back of a chair for support.

## **the payoff:**

Defines your inner thighs—beautiful!

**sets -n- reps:** Do three sets of 20 to 25 reps.
**must-haves:** Nada

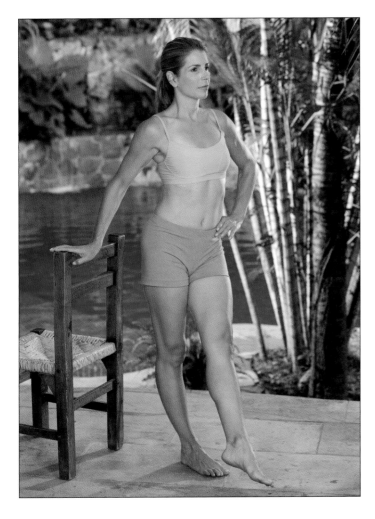

**POSITION 1:** Lift your left leg across your body so the heel of your foot sweeps past your standing foot. Do 20 to 25 reps.

## FABULOUS FORM TIPS

○ Don't lift your leg too high. It's all about the ultra-squeeze in your inner thighs.

○ Don't move your hips. Keep your abs turned on to help stabilize your hips while your leg moves.

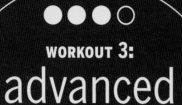

**WORKOUT 3:**
# advanced

inner thigh circles
with ankle weights

hydrant inner thigh with
3-pound ball

scissor legs stationary
with leg weights

---

**THE PAYOFF:**
## Slenderizes your
## inner thighs!

---

**TOTAL TIME:** 15 to 20 minutes

**HOW OFTEN:** Remember, squeeze, engage,
and focus, and slimtastic is no longer a dream.
Breathe normally. Do this workout three times a
week on nonconsecutive days.

★ **RESIZE YOUR THIGHS,**
**on page 100, offers more advice**
**for maximizing this workout.**

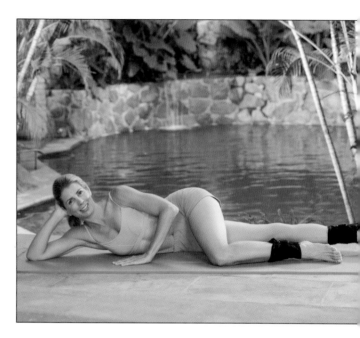

**STARTING POSITION:** Wrap an ankle weight around
each ankle and then lie on your right side with your left
leg bent over your right. Prop your head on your right
arm. Inhale to lift your top leg about hip height.

## the payoff:
Strong and sexy inner thighs!

# with ankle weights

**sets -n- reps:** Do three sets of 25 to 30 reps.
**must-haves:** Pair of 5-pound (2-kg) ankle weights

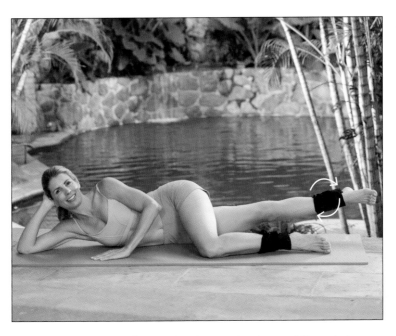

**POSITION 1:** Lift your bottom leg to your top leg and then circle it, engaging your inner thighs (try touching 'em together) on each circle. Do 25 to 30 circles.

## FABULOUS FORM TIPS

○ Don't lift from your foot. Instead, lift from your knee all the way up to fire up your inner thighs.

○ Use your inner thighs when circling your leg; imagine your inner thighs are kissing.

# **3** hydrant inner thigh with 3-pound ball

○○○○

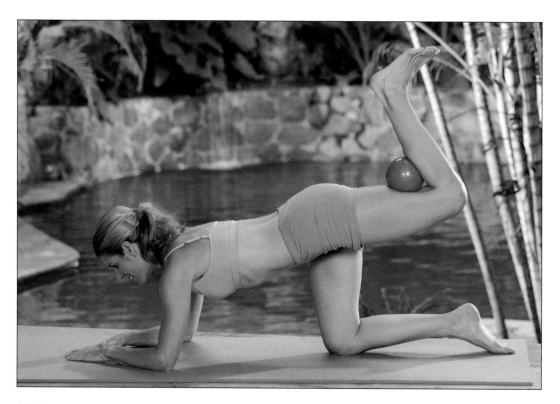

**STARTING POSITION:** Place your knees and elbows on the floor. Place a 3-pound (1.5-kg) ball behind your left knee. Relax your head, neck, and shoulders and look down. Lift your left leg up, leading with your heel as if you're making an imprint of your foot on the ceiling. Squeeze your booty as you lift your leg so your knee is in line with your hipbones.

## **the payoff:**
Slims your inner thighs and gets your butt too!

**sets -n- reps:**   Do three sets of 25 to 30 reps.
**must-haves:**   3-pound (1.5-kg) ball

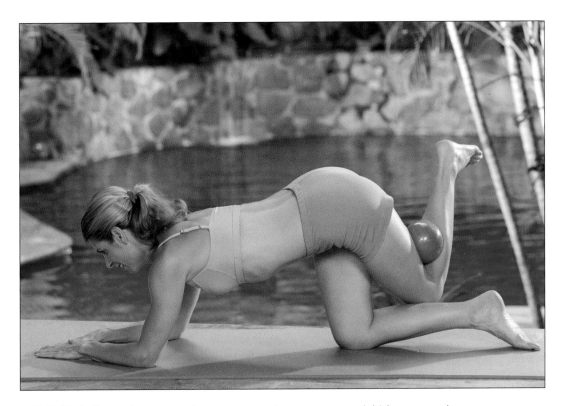

**POSITION 1:** As you lower your leg, cross your knee over your right leg, squeezing your inner thighs scary-tight until you feel the contraction between your thighs. Do 25 to 30 reps.

## FABULOUS FORM TIPS

❍ Don't forget that the focus is *lowering your leg* and squeezing your inner thighs.

❍ Don't lift your knee too high; otherwise, you may feel strain in your lower back.

❍ Use your booty to get some extra rear work, pushing to the point of a full-on contraction.

❍ Use your abs to help stabilize your belly. Lift your belly button to your spine the whole time.

❍ Use oh-so-small controlled movements to isolate your inner thighs!

# **3** scissor legs with leg weights

○○○○

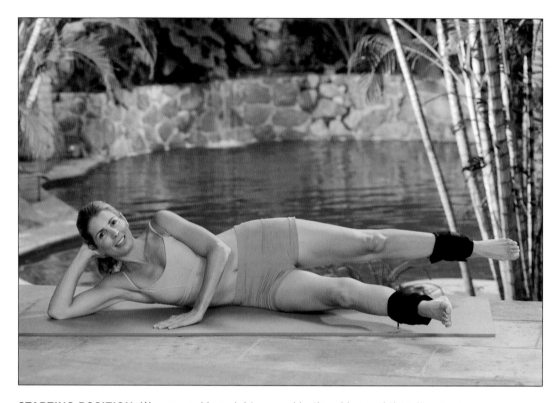

**STARTING POSITION:** Wrap an ankle weight around both ankles and then lie on your right side with your legs straight, ankles, knees, and hipbones stacked on top of one another and your feet parallel. Prop up your head on your right arm. Lift both legs off the floor. Open your legs like a pair of scissors.

## **the payoff:**

Slenderizes your legs lean!

**sets -n- reps:**   Do three sets of 25 to 30 reps.
**must-haves:**   Pair of 5-pound (2-kg) ankle weights

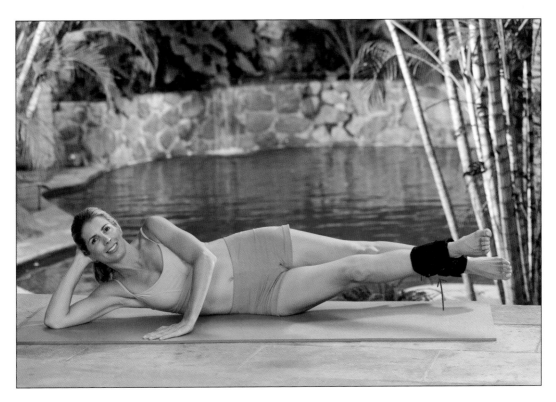

**POSITION 1:** Hold your scissors and lift your bottom leg, as if your inner thighs were kissing, and then lower it. Do 25 to 30 reps.

## FABULOUS FORM TIPS

○  Don't move your legs as you lift the bottom leg up; lifts are not big because the focus is on both legs squeezing together.

○  Use your abs to stabilize your hips so you can isolate and work those inner thighs.

○  Don't worry if you feel your outer thigh heating up. You *abso* should!

○●●● ●

**WORKOUT 4:**

# super advanced

v squeeze with ball
big ball beats
anding adduction leg lift
with ankle weights

---

**THE PAYOFF:**
Melts your
inner thigh flab!

---

**TOTAL TIME:** 15 to 20 minutes

**HOW OFTEN:** Let the slim thighs roll;
it's all about this moment and the work you've
been doing up to now, so keep going!
Breathe normally. Do this workout three times
a week on nonconsecutive days.

★ **RESIZE YOUR THIGHS,**
on page 100, offers more advice
for maximizing this workout.

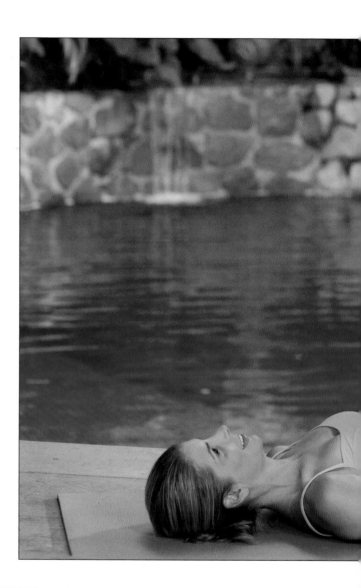

## the payoff:

Squeeze your heart out to
lean those thighs!

# ball

**sets -n- reps:** Do three sets of at least 25 to 30 reps.
**must-haves:** Stability ball

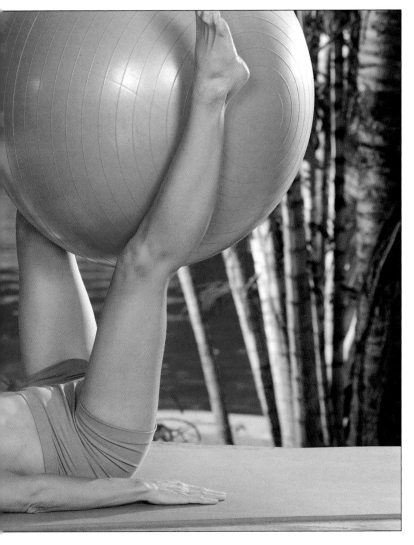

**STARTING POSITION:** Lie on your back with straight legs and place your stability ball between your legs. Lay your arms by your sides.

**POSITION 1:** Squeeze your thighs and release, squeeze and release. Do *lotsa* reps, at least 25 to 30.

## FABULOUS FORM TIPS

○ Don't forget that the focus is on your inner thighs.

○ Squeeze from your knees and all the way up.

# **4** big ball beats

○○○○

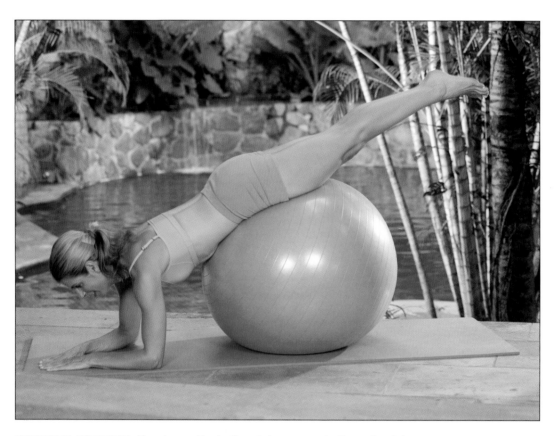

**STARTING POSITION:** Kneel over the ball and drape your belly and pelvis over the ball. Roll on your hips so the ball supports your torso. Place your elbows on the floor in front of the ball. Gaze at the floor. Lift your legs, engaging your glutes, with your heels together.

## the payoff:

Melts your inner thigh flab!

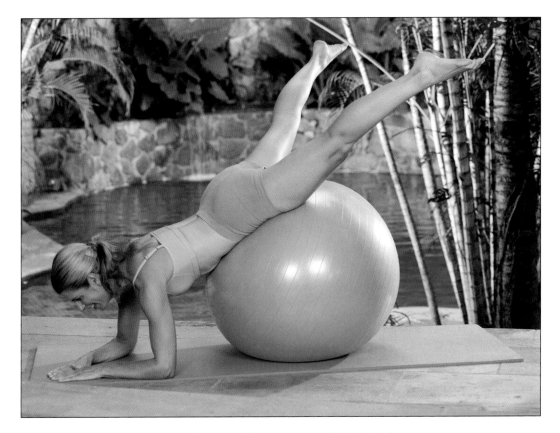

**POSITION 1:** Inhale to open your legs as wide as you can. Exhale to close your legs, engaging your inner thighs (tons of booty work, too). Do many reps, 25 to 30. If you need a rest, drape yourself over the ball after you're done and just breathe. It's a yummy lower back stretch.

## FABULOUS FORM TIPS

○ Don't sag your belly; lift your belly button to your spine the whole time to give your lower back support.

○ Don't forget to firm up your fanny; put a thousand-dollar bill between your butt cheeks—well, at least imagine it!

# **4** standing adduction leg lifts with ankle

○○○○

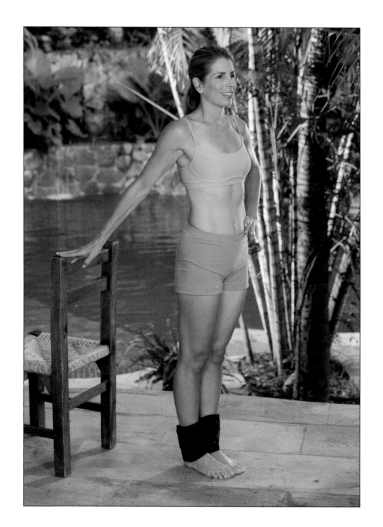

**STARTING POSITION:** Wrap a 5-pound (2-kg) ankle weight around each ankle. Stand with your feet together, parallel with each other, and straighten your arms by your sides. Your hip points should face forward and remain even. Lift from the top of your head and drop your shoulders. Place your fingertips on a wall or hold the back of a chair for support.

## **the payoff:**

Bye-bye inner thigh flappage!

# weights

| | |
|---|---|
| **sets -n- reps:** | Do three sets of at least 25 to 30 reps. |
| **must-haves:** | Pair of 5-pound (2-kg) ankle weights |

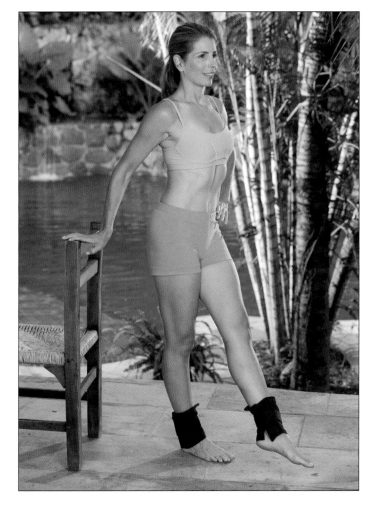

**POSITION 1:** Lift your left leg across your body so the heel of your foot sweeps past your standing foot and then return to the starting position, but don't touch the floor. Do *lotsa* reps—at least 25 to 30.

## FABULOUS FORM TIPS

❍ Don't lift your leg too high. It's about the ultra squeeze in your inner thighs.

❍ Don't move your hips. Keep your abs turned on to help stabilize your hips while your leg moves.

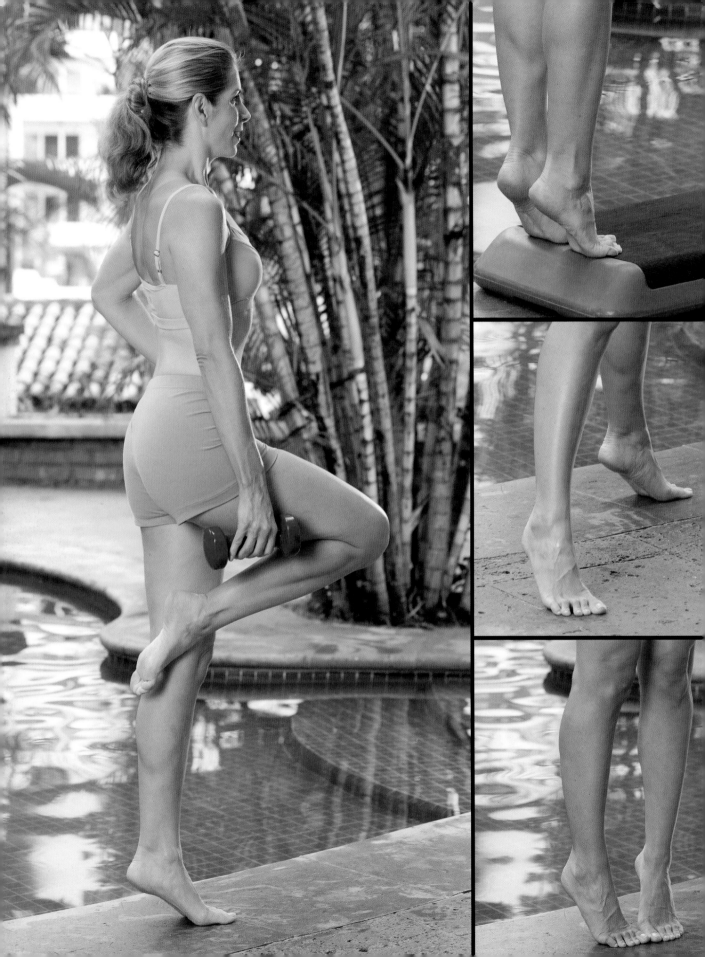

# chapter 7

# CANKLES, BEGONE!

| | | the payoff | total time | how often | sets -n- reps | must-haves |
|---|---|---|---|---|---|---|
| **WORKOUT 1–2:** ⭕⭕⭕⭕ ⭕⭕⭕⭕<br>beginner to intermediate<br><br>Calf Raise in Parallel<br>Calf Raise (Toes In)<br>Calf Raise (Toes Out) | | Shapes your calves— lovely in your stilettos! | 10 minutes | Do this workout 3 times a week on non-consecutive days, such as Mon., Wed., and Fri. | Do three sets of 8 to 15 reps. | Pair of 3- to 5-pound (1.5- to 2-kg) dumbbells |
| **WORKOUT 3–4:** ⭕⭕⭕⭕ ⭕⭕⭕⭕<br>advanced to super advanced<br><br>Calf Raise in Parallel (Platform)<br>Calf Raise (Single Leg)<br>Squat with Calf Raise<br>Plié Squat with Calf Raise | | Sculpts 'em really sexy! | 10 to 15 minutes | Do this workout 3 times a week on non-consecutive days, such as Mon., Wed., and Fri. | Do three sets of 15 to 20 reps. | 3- to 5-pound (1.5- to 2-kg) dumbbell and a step |

# beginner to intermediate

calf raise in parallel
calf raise (toes in)
calf raise (toes out)

---

**THE PAYOFF:**
## Shapes your calves— lovely in your stilettos!

---

**TOTAL TIME:** 10 minutes

**HOW OFTEN:** Spend two to four weeks building good overall strength in your calves. Try these exercises first without the dumbbells. If they're too easy, add the extra weight. Do this workout three times a week on nonconsecutive days.

★ **SHAPE YOUR ANKLES,**
on page 101, offers more advice
for maximizing this workout.

# 1-2 calf raise in
○○○○
○○○○

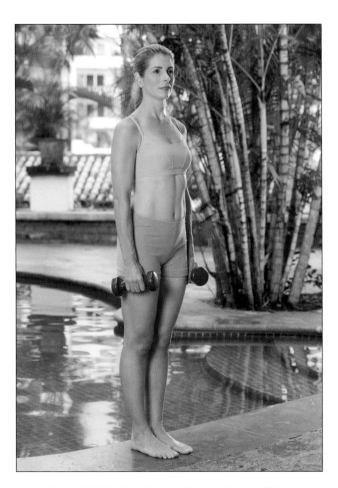

**STARTING POSITION:** Stand with your feet a little wider than hip-width apart, with your toes pointing straight ahead. Hold a dumbbell in each hand. Look forward and slightly up.

## the payoff:

Carves out crazy-hot calves!

# parallel

**sets -n- reps:** Do three sets of 8 to 15 reps.
**must-haves:** Pair of 3- to 5-pound (1.5- to 2-kg) dumbbells

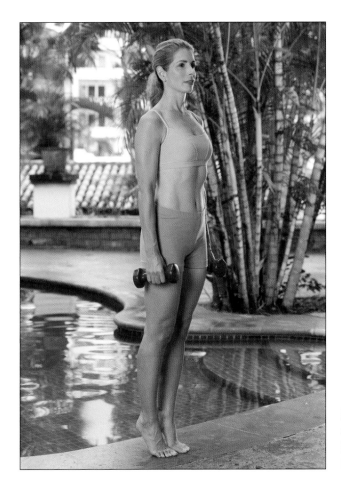

**POSITION 1:** Lift your heels off the floor. Keep your chest lifted and your spine straight, with all of your body weight evenly placed between your big and little toes. Do 8 to 15 reps.

## FABULOUS FORM TIPS

❍ Engage your abs to help you balance.

❍ Focus on raising up evenly in your foot to build good overall strength.

# 1-2  calf raise (toes in)

○○○○
○○○○

**sets -n- reps:** Do three sets of 8 to 15 reps.

**must-haves:** Pair of 3- to 5-pound (1.5- to 2-kg) dumbbells

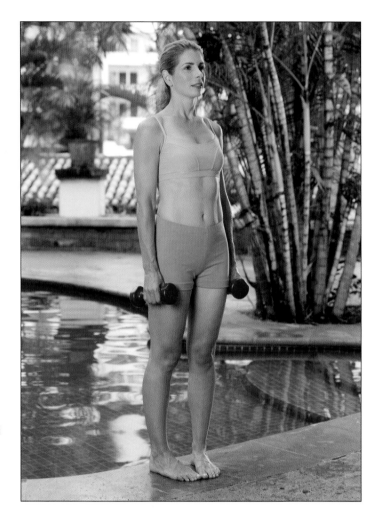

**STARTING POSITION:** Stand with your feet a little wider than hip-width apart and turn your toes in, making about a 6-inch (15 cm) gap between your heels. Hold a dumbbell in each hand. Look forward and slightly up.

## the payoff:

Shapes your calves—especially your outer calves!

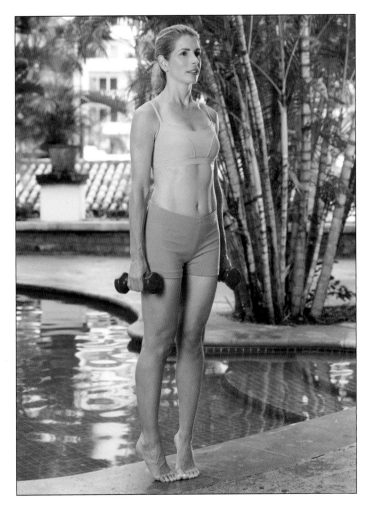

**POSITION 1:** Lift your heels off the floor. Keep your chest lifted and your spine straight, with all of your body weight evenly placed between your big and little toes. Do 8 to 15 reps.

## FABULOUS FORM TIPS

- Engage your abs to help you balance. You may feel wobbly in this position, so be careful.

- Focus on raising up evenly in your foot to shape your outer calves.

- Focus on putting pressure on the big and little toes.

# 1-2 calf raise (toes out)

○○○○
○○○○

**sets -n- reps:** Do three sets of 8 to 15 reps.
**must-haves:** Pair of 3- to 5-pound (1.5- to 2-kg) dumbbells

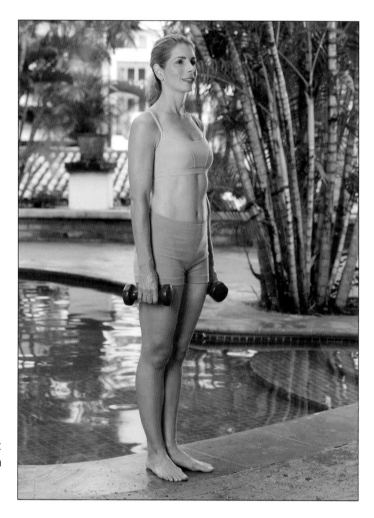

**STARTING POSITION:** Stand with your feet turned out so that your heels touch. Hold a dumbbell in each hand. Look forward and slightly up.

## the payoff:

Shapes your calves—especially your inner calves

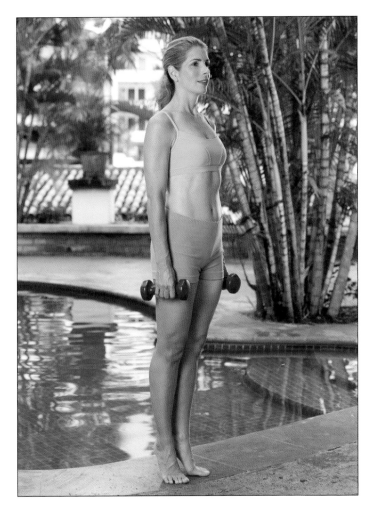

**POSITION 1:** Lift your heels off the floor. Keep your chest lifted and your spine straight, with all of your body weight evenly placed between your big and little toes. Do 8 to 15 reps.

## FABULOUS FORM TIPS

○ Engage your abs to help you balance.

○ Keep your heels together, and you'll get a little extra inner thigh work.

○ Focus on lifting up evenly in your foot to build overall strength and beauty.

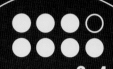

**WORKOUT 3–4:**

# advanced to super advanced

calf raise in parallel (platform)
calf raise (single leg)
squat with calf raise
plié squat with
calf raise

**THE PAYOFF:**
Sculpts 'em really sexy!

**TOTAL TIME:** 10 to 15 minutes

**HOW OFTEN:** Now, spend two to four weeks to sculpt your calves sexy. Do this workout three times a week on nonconsecutive days.

★ **SHAPE YOUR ANKLES,**
on page 101, offers more advice
for maximizing this workout.

# 3–4 calf raise in

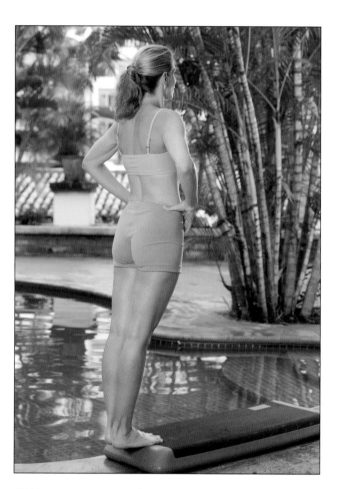

**STARTING POSITION:** Step up on a platform with your feet hip-width apart, toes pointing straight ahead. Look forward and slightly up.

## the payoff:
Lovely lower legs!

# parallel (platform)

**sets -n- reps:** Do three sets of 15 to 20 reps.

**must-haves:** A step platform (one riser) or stand off your steps at home

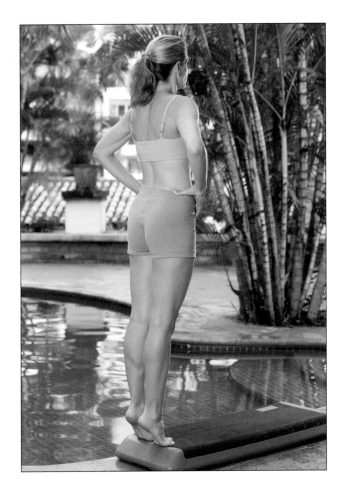

**POSITION 1:** Lift your heels up. Keep your chest lifted and your spine straight, with all of your body weight evenly placed between your big and little toes. Do 15 to 20 reps.

## FABULOUS FORM TIPS

- ○ Engage your abs to help you balance.

- ○ Focus on lifting up evenly in your foot to build good overall strength.

- ○ To increase the intensity, hold a dumbbell in each hand.

# 3-4 calf raise (single leg)

○○○○
○○○○

**sets -n- reps:** Do three sets of 15 to 20 reps.
**must-haves:** 3- to 5-pound (1.5- to 2-kg) dumbbells

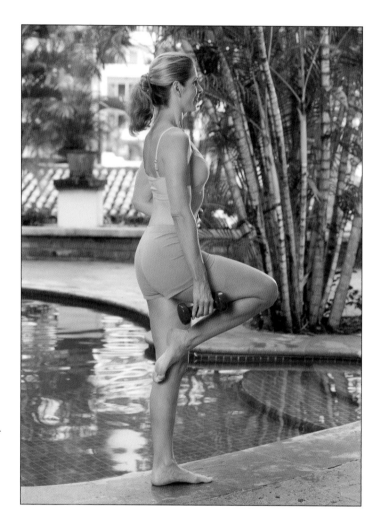

**STARTING POSITION:** Stand with your feet a little wider than hip-width apart, toes pointing straight ahead. Bend your right knee and hold a dumbbell in your right hand. If you need support, hold a wall with your left hand. Look forward and slightly up.

## the payoff:
Strengthens your calves!

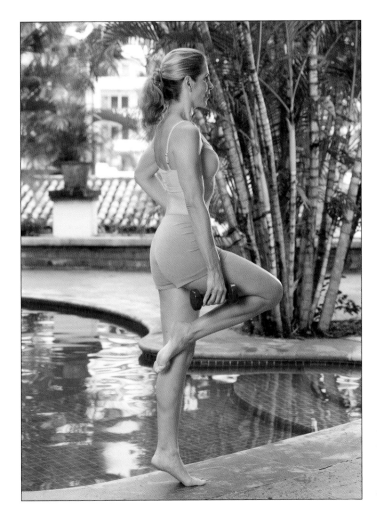

**POSITION 1:** Stand on your tiptoes and then lower to your heel. Keep your chest lifted and your spine straight, with all of your body weight evenly placed between your big and little toes. Do 15 to 20 reps.

## FABULOUS FORM TIPS

○ Engage your abs to help you balance.

○ Use a light touch when holding the wall to challenge your balance.

○ Focus on rising up evenly in your foot to build overall strength and beauty.

# 3-4 squat with calf raise

○○○○
○○○○

**sets -n- reps:** Do three sets of 15 to 20 reps.
**must-haves:** Nothing

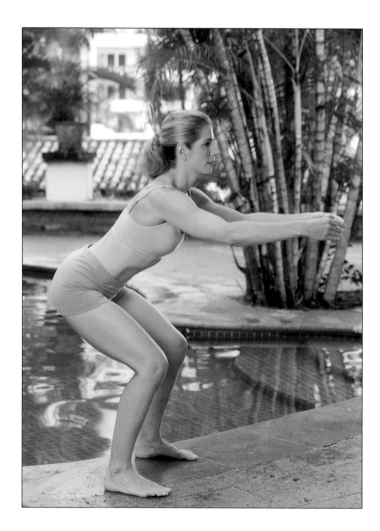

**STARTING POSITION:** Stand with your feet hip-width apart. Look forward and slightly up. Lower your bottom only until your thighs are parallel to the floor, knees aligned with the second and third toes. Keep your chest lifted and your spine straight, with the majority of your body weight in your heels.

## the payoff:

Gives you great gams!

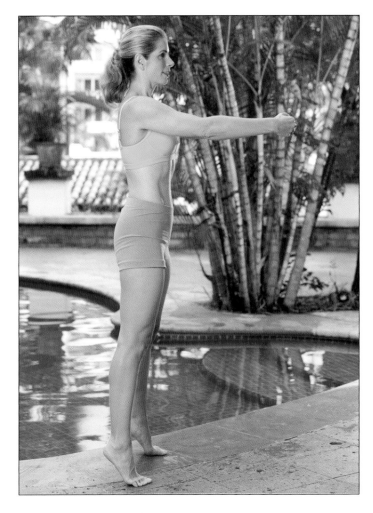

**POSITION 1:** As you come up, lift up on your tiptoes. Do 15 to 20 reps.

## FABULOUS FORM TIPS

- Don't lean forward. Your torso will naturally come forward slightly as you squat.

- Don't turn your knees in. Keep them stable and point your toes forward as you squat down.

- Use sexy posture. Straighten your spine from the top of your head and down and relax your shoulders.

- Turn on your abs to balance as you lift to work the calves, and hold the lift for a second.

- Focus on lifting up evenly in your foot to build beautiful calves.

# 3-4 plié squat with calf raise

○○○○
○○○○

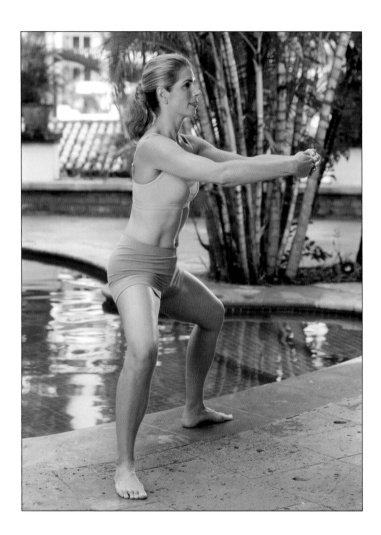

**STARTING POSITION:** Stand with your feet about 3 feet apart (twice hip-width), and turn out your toes. Look forward and slightly up. Lower your bottom only until your thighs are parallel to the floor, with your knees aligned with your second and third toes. Keep your chest lifted and your spine straight, with the majority of your body weight in your heels.

## the payoff:

Works the leg sexy!

**sets -n- reps:** Do three sets of 15 to 20 reps.
**must-haves:** Nothing

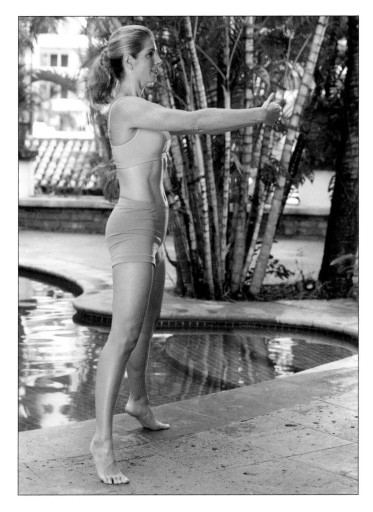

**POSITION 1:** As you come up, lift up on your tiptoes. Do 15 to 20 reps.

## FABULOUS FORM TIPS

- ○ Don't turn your knees in. Focus on putting the majority of your body weight on the outside edges of your feet.

- ○ Don't forget to squeeze your bottom when you lift up for major underbutt and inner thigh benefits.

- ○ Use sexy posture. Straighten your spine from the top of your head and down and relax your shoulders.

- ○ Use your abs to balance as you lift up on your tiptoes.

- ○ Hold dumbells to increase intensity.

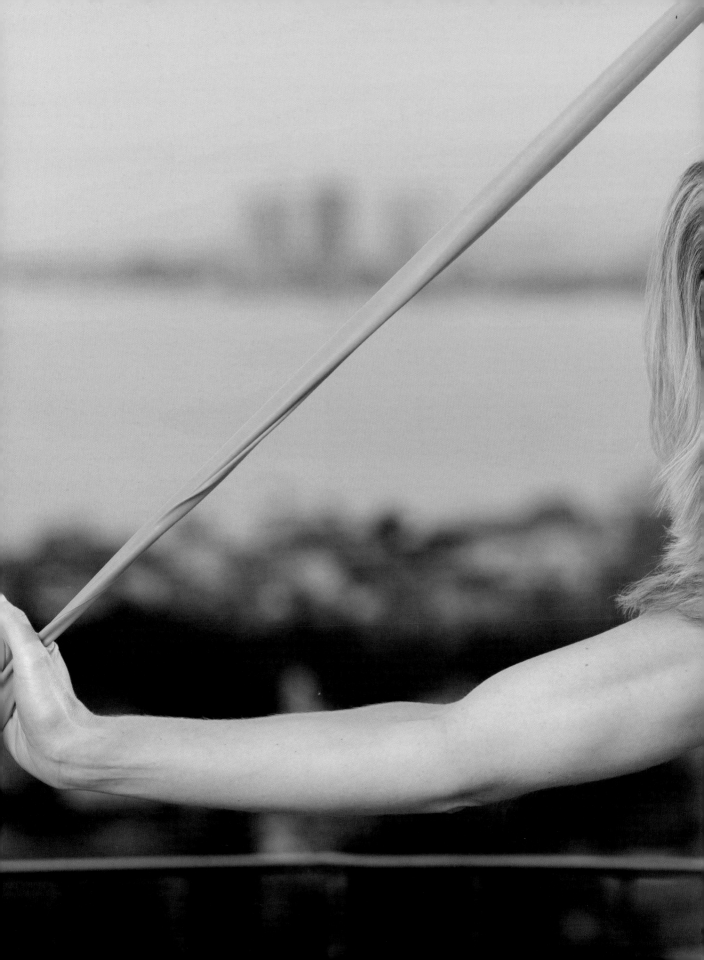

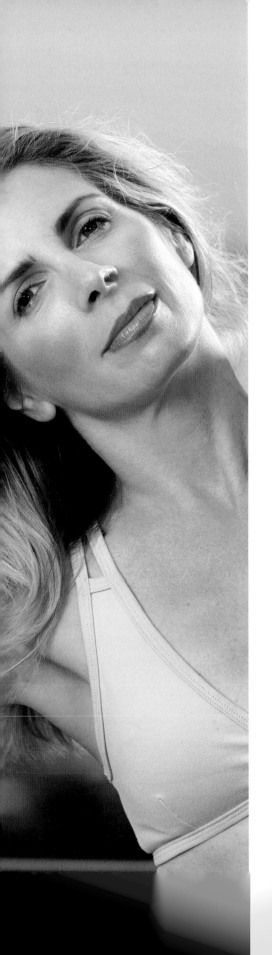

 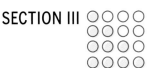

# The Best Upper Body Workouts

### you'll be hot to trot in your tank top!

**Every little sexy curve** you sculpt now—on your shoulders, back, chest, and arms—will show in your tank top, halter dress, or bikini. So work it out, and say au revoir to flabby arms, slouchy shoulders, and back fat! Day by day these exercises will sculpt you—c'est va-va-voom!—with workouts that target the following areas.

Get ready to strut your sexy stuff!

# Say Yes to Skinny Success: My Favorite Tips

**Start in the kitchen.** I've said it before: skinny starts right in your own kitchen. Don't buy foods that sabotage your hot bod! In other words, if you don't buy it, you won't eat it, and chances are your family members don't need it, either.

**Slim down with water.** The best thing that I do consistently every day is drink lots of water, specifically 1 quart (liter) first thing in the morning, a quart (liter)-plus after exercise, and then another one throughout my day. Focus on eating foods that are high in water, too, such as soups loaded with veggies and your favorite fruits, both of which can fill you up faster and help prevent you from overindulging. Big bonus: your skin will look lovely.

**Say bah-bye to bad fats:** Avoid all trans fats, which studies show can pack on the pounds and harm your heart! Trans fats are found in vegetable shortenings, margarines, vending-machine foods such as cookies and crackers, snack foods, and fast foods.

**Break your fast.** Eating first thing ignites your calorie-burning engine and helps prevent you from overeating all day. You can be creative here. Three of my favorite 2-minute breakfasts are nonfat plain yogurt, blueberries, and walnuts; multigrain toast with banana and yummy almond butter; and a bowl of healthful high-fiber cereal, nonfat milk, and fruit.

**Sample sweets sparingly.** Yes, you can have chocolate and other temptations. Just make sure that these foods give you a little something back—such as nutrients! By eating dark chocolate, you get precious antioxidants. Nuts give you heart-healthy fats and omega-3s, such as walnuts. Just eat them both in moderation. My personal favorite sweets are Fig Newmans (Paul Newman's brand of the traditional favorites) because they're so yummy and packed with fiber.

**Pleeease eat carbs.** To keep you going throughout your day, eat gritty and grainy carbs. Look for ones that contain whole wheat, multigrains, bran, or rye. Research shows that the more fiber in your diet, the skinnier and healthier you are because fiber fills you up, causing you to eat less of the bad stuff. Eat your carbs for breakfast and have some at lunch but shoot for none at dinner. (Ditch the bread basket.) No white anything—flour, breads, or rice.

**Don't have food meltdowns.** Don't come unglued if you have a little Ben and Jerry's. It's just not realistic to eat perfectly every day. Allow a day for a little wiggle room—perhaps on the day you take a break from exercise. This allowance makes it so much more rewarding (and easier) to eat well and exercise on the days you should be exercising.

# Sculpt and Scorch the Calories with Cardio

To lose fat and tone your muscles, you'll do a cardio session on the treadmill, holding a pair of 2- or 3-pound (1- or 1.5-kg) dumbbells for your arms. Each session lasts about 50 minutes. You'll have a choice between two treadmill workouts. In Sculpting Workout One, you'll hold a pair of dumbbells to shape your arms and walk on the treadmill (great for beginners), while in Sculpting Workout Two, you'll walk on an incline while holding a pair of dumbbells.

Don't fret about the dumbbells. It's simple to hold a dumbbell in each hand, palms up, elbows bent and by your sides, moving your arms like you're walking really fast. In fact, you'll actually be walking fast, so follow the directions below and flab will sooo melt.

Here's a warning: if you have a shoulder injury, holding a pair of dumbbells may not be right for you. When in doubt, always check with your health care practitioner.

If you hate the treadmill, try the elliptical machine and work your arms, too! You can do this workout outside; just don't forget your dumbbells. Pick your workout and do it four times a week.

## Sculpting Workout One

This workout should take 50 minutes.

**4 minutes:** Warm up by walking 3.2 mph to 3.5 mph, no grade
**46 minutes:** Walk 3.8 mph to 4.0 mph, no grade
**2 minutes:** Cool down by walking 3.2 to 3.5, no grade

## Sculpting Workout Two

This workout is more challenging because it adds an incline.

**4 minutes:** Warm up by walking 3.2 to 3.5 mph, no grade
**4 minutes:** Walk 3.8 to 4.0 mph, 3 percent grade (breathless pace)
**2 minutes:** Walk 3.8 to 4.0 mph, 5 percent grade (break-a-sweat pace)

### INTERVAL ONE
**8 minutes:** Walk 3.8 to 4.0 mph, 3 percent grade (breathless pace)
**2 minutes:** Walk 3.8 to 4.0 mph, 5 percent grade (break-a-sweat pace)

### INTERVAL TWO
**8 minutes:** Walk 3.8 to 4.0 mph, 3 percent grade (breathless pace).
**2 minutes:** Walk 3.8 to 4.0 mph, 5 percent grade (break-a-sweat pace)

### INTERVAL THREE
**8 minutes:** Walk 3.8 to 4.0 mph, 3 percent grade (breathless pace)
**2 minutes:** Walk 3.8 to 4.0 mph, 5 percent grade (break-a-sweat pace)

### INTERVAL FOUR
**8 minutes:** Walk 3.8 to 4.0 mph, 3 percent grade (breathless pace)
**2 minutes:** Walk 3.8 to 4.0 mph, 5 percent grade (break-a-sweat pace)
**2 minutes:** Cool down by walking 2 minutes at 3.2 to 3.5, no grade

# Getting to Know Your Muscles

Let's start by getting to know your back muscles. Strong back muscles are so sexy, and they're so important to your overall health. What's not sexy is chronic back pain. Your best chance to avoid both back pain and back injury is to maintain good, overall back strength. So focus on your deepest back muscle, called the **multifidus**, because it works around the clock to stabilize and support your spine to keep your spine healthy.

Sitting on top of your multifidus are your **erector spinae**, or spinal erectors. Collectively, these muscles run the length of your spine and help keep your back straight. Just about every exercise or sport calls on these muscles, so it's important to keep them fit and strong.

On your upper back are a variety of muscles. Some of the heavy hitters are your **trapezius**, or traps, which form a diamond-shaped muscle originating on the base of the skull, attaching the shoulder blades, and ending around the middle of your back. It's your traps that assist in lowering and lifting your shoulders. (We're going to focus on strengthening the lower traps, which are located in your midback or your bra line.)

Sitting between your shoulder blades are the rhomboids, which help stabilize your shoulder blades and draw your shoulder blades together to open your chest.

Then there is the **serratus anterior**, which is a thin muscle that originates on your lateral ribs and connects under your shoulder blades. This muscle also helps stabilize your shoulder blades to keep them flat on your back while keeping your shoulders in place.

The biggest back muscle is the **latissimus dorsi**, or your lats. It fans across your back, extending from the lower spine to the upper arm bone, and is pretty superficial. In fact, you can feel it working in most exercises.

Your chest muscles, or **pectoralis minor** and **pectoralis major**, form a broad band across your chest and are super important in the posture department. When these muscles are tight, the opposing muscles on your back lengthen and get weak. Sounds like a bad recipe for slumped, slouchy shoulders. Of course, you don't want this to happen because it's not sexy, and over time you may alter the bones of your upper back, potentially causing an ugly hump in your midback.

Your shoulder muscles are called your **deltoids**, or delts, and are divided into three parts to support your shoulders: anterior, or front portion of your shoulder; middle, which sits on top of your shoulder; and posterior, or back shoulder. Imagine a helmet sitting on top, covering and protecting your shoulder bones. Sitting underneath your delts are the very delicate **rotator cuff muscles**, which primarily help stabilize your shoulders and prevent dislocation of the shoulder joint.

You'll focus on two muscles to get your beautiful arms—your triceps and biceps. Your **triceps** are located on the back of your arm and tend to be

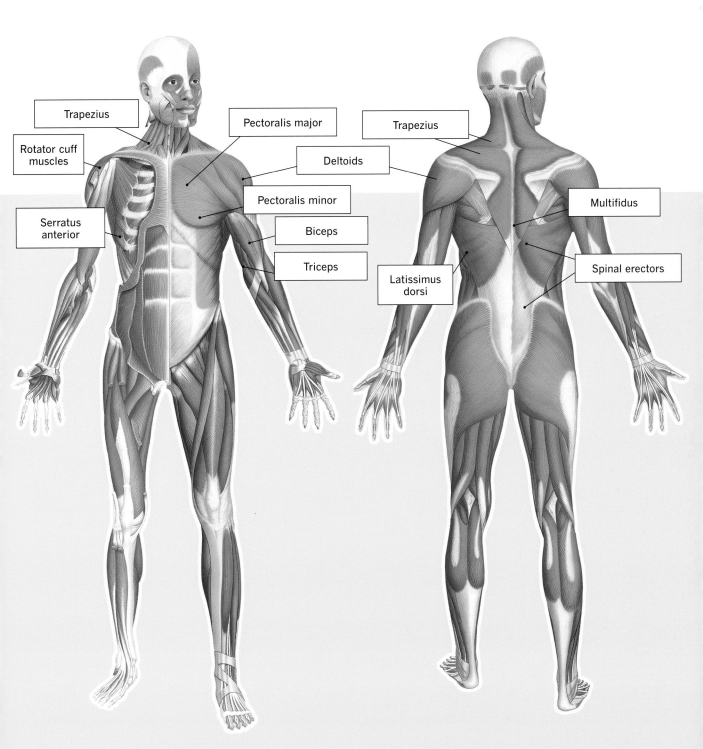

Trapezius

Rotator cuff muscles

Serratus anterior

Pectoralis major

Deltoids

Pectoralis minor

Biceps

Triceps

Trapezius

Multifidus

Spinal erectors

Latissimus dorsi

every woman's nightmare. Because the triceps are hard to tone and are often cursed with loose skin, you'll do lots of exercises for 'em.

Your **biceps**, on the other hand, located on the front of the arm, usually get plenty of work throughout your day and stay pretty toned. In these workouts, you'll work the triceps in a variety of angles to stimulate all the muscle fibers, plus you'll hit your biceps, too.

# Maximize Your Upper Body Work

## PERFECT YOUR POSTURE
Try these tips to get great posture.

★ **Move your pits to your hips.** Drop your shoulders away from your ears and never do these exercises with your shoulders lifted to your ears.

★ **Get in touch with your bra line**. Probably some of the weakest muscles on your body are in your midback; isolating these muscles is hard because the upper traps always want to come into action. Try to feel the work in your midback.

★ **Don't get a belly pooch.** Because you'll be prone, or facedown, doing most of these exercises, you may forget about your belly. Never, ladies! Your belly supports your lower back and provides toning benefits, so lift your belly button to your spine the whole time so you don't stress your lower back.

★ **Make micro movements.** Because most of this work focuses on delicate back muscles, move in itsy-bitsy amounts to properly engage working muscles.

★ **Keep your pelvis perfect.** Don't move your pelvis in these exercises. Instead, keep it stable and work in a neutral pelvis. (See page 11.)

★ **Breathe.** These exercises all have directions on how to breathe, but if you get stuck, just remember this: always inhale to move into an extension or to arch your back and lift your chest off the mat.

## BEAUTIFUL-BACK BASICS
Take note, girls: two things must happen for a beautiful back. First, you need to gain awareness in how you hold your shoulders throughout the day, and second, you need to build strength in the muscles that support good posture.

From this point on, do this trick: lift your shoulders to your ears, gently bring 'em back (not too far) and then slide your shoulder blades down your back to drop your shoulders away from your ears, or pits to hips.

This movement requires a variety of muscles surrounding the two winged bones on your back (your shoulder blades). These bones are important because they stabilize your shoulder girdle. When the muscles surrounding these bones are strong, your upper back is far healthier and can better support good posture. Slumped shoulders are not pretty (for sure), but consider the other crazy-scary things that could happen in your body: you can lose an inch or more in your height, your breathing may be compromised as your rib cage compresses your lungs, your neck looks squatty, your chest drops (you may lose a cup size), and you may get constant headaches and back pain.

Use the photos on the opposite page to practice un-rounding your shoulders.

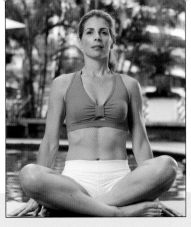
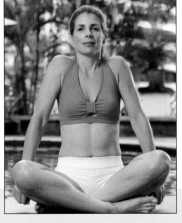

Left: Lift your shoulders up and back and down slightly to perfect your posture. Engage the muscles underneath your armpits by imagining putting a couple of pencils between your ribs and upper arms—now squeeze.

Right: Urgh, working with lifted shoulders by your ears is sooo not sexy!

In truth, if you haven't been aware of how you hold your shoulders, standing tall will take some time. It may be difficult because over time the muscles on your upper back weaken, getting too long to support good posture, while the muscles on the front of your body get very tight. But that's where these exercises come in.

## GET A NATURAL LIFT

Keep the following tips in mind as you do each of the exercises in chapter 9.

★ **Focus and squeeze.** To work your chest muscles, actively squeeze your chest as you work to isolate these muscles.

★ **Don't let your belly sag.** Focus on lifting your belly button to your spine the whole time, especially as you do, let's say, push-ups.

★ **Shoulders down.** Don't lift your shoulders to your ears.

## SCULPTED SEXY SHOULDER TIPS

And use the following advice in chapter 10.

★ **Go easy.** Most upper body exercises include your shoulders, which can easily fatigue them. So don't forget to drop your shoulders away from your ears; otherwise, you may overwork them and then they may not respond to the work you're about to do!

★ **Use proper form.** Relax your chest so it won't take over for your delts. If you feel your chest rise, focus on good posture, making your back straight or flush with a bench.

★ **Keep your head straight.** Don't turn your head; keep it in line with your spine.

## AMAZING ARM TIPS

Use these tips for the exercises in chapter 11.

★ **Don't use momentum.** Don't swing your arms through the work. Instead, focus and squeeze to get the most work out of your muscles.

★ **Don't have a belly bulge.** Just because you're focusing on your arms doesn't mean you should let your belly pooch. Engage your abs, too!

★ **Keep your shoulders down.** Drop your shoulders to your ears to isolate the work in your arms.

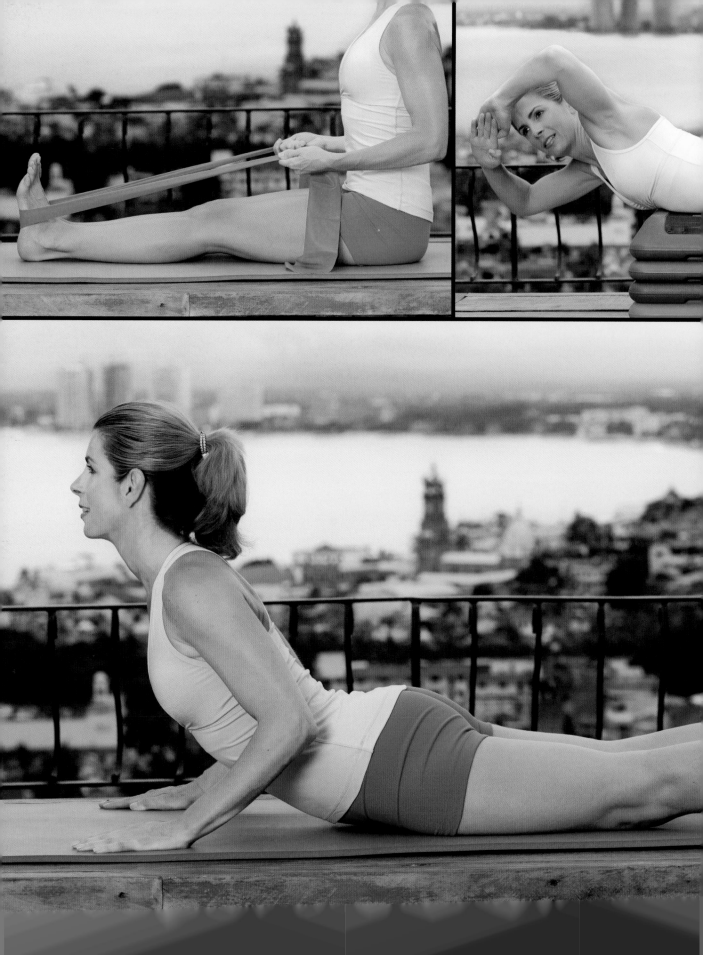

# chapter 8

# POSTURE PERFECT

| | | the payoff | total time | how often | sets -n- reps | must-haves |
|---|---|---|---|---|---|---|
| **WORKOUT 1:**<br>beginner<br><br>Multifidus Deep Back Work<br>Flight<br>Single-Leg Hip Extension | ○○○○ | Strengthens your back beautiful! | 15 to 20 minutes | Do this workout 3 times a week on non-consecutive days, such as Mon., Wed., and Fri. | Do three sets of 5 reps. | Nothing |
| **WORKOUT 2:**<br>intermediate<br><br>Cobra<br>Cross Extension<br>Row with Resistance Band | ○○○○ | Lengthens your look (Wouldn't you want that?) | 15 to 20 minutes | Do this workout 3 times a week on non-consecutive days, such as Mon., Wed., and Fri. | Do three sets of the number of reps given in each exercise. | Resistance band |
| **WORKOUT 3:**<br>advanced<br><br>Snorkel<br>Snorkel with Goalpost Arms<br>Lift and Rotate (Extension) | ○○○○ | Perfects your posture, hot stuff! | 15 to 20 minutes | Do this workout 3 times a week on non-consecutive days, such as Mon., Wed., and Fri. | Do three sets of the number of reps given in each exercise. | Step or bench |
| **WORKOUT 4:**<br>super advanced<br><br>Snorkel with Big Ball<br>Lift and Rotate with Big Ball<br>Single-Leg Bent-Over Row | ○○○○ | Beats the back fat! | 15 to 20 minutes | Do this workout 3 times a week on non-consecutive days, such as Mon., Wed., and Fri. | Do three sets of the number of reps given in each exercise. | Stability ball, a pair of 5- to 10-pound (2- to 4.5-kg) dumbbells, and a step or bench |

○○○○ **WORKOUT 1:**

# beginner

multifidus deep back work
flight
single-leg hip extension

---

**THE PAYOFF:**
## Strengthens your back beautiful!

---

**TOTAL TIME:** 15 to 20 minutes

**HOW OFTEN:** Spend two to four weeks building strength in your back muscles. Now is the time to nail down good form so you don't stress out your lower back. Here's a warning: if you have a back injury, ask your doctor before trying these exercises. Do this workout three times a week on nonconsecutive days.

★ **PERFECT YOUR POSTURE,**
on page 202, offers more advice for maximizing this workout.

**1** ○○○○
# multifidus deep back work

| | |
|---|---|
| **sets -n- reps:** | Do three sets of 5 reps. |
| **must-haves:** | Nothing |

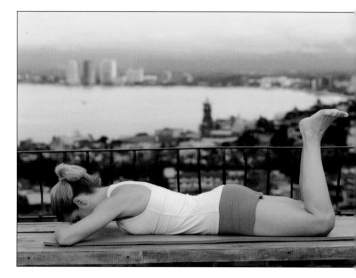

**STARTING POSITION:** Lie on your stomach with your knees bent and put your heels together so your legs make the shape of a diamond. Rest your arms over your head, crossing your hands to rest your head on top of your hands, palms down. Press your heels together as if you have a dime between your heels. Squeeze and release, focusing on lifting your belly button to your spine the whole time. Do 5 reps.

## the payoff:
Builds an unbeatable lower back

# 1 flight

○○○○

**sets -n- reps:** Do three sets of 5 reps.
**must-haves:** Nothing

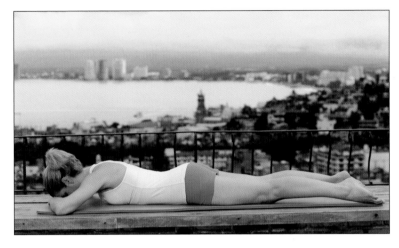

**STARTING POSITION:** Lie on your stomach with your legs straight and place your hands under your forehead, palms down.

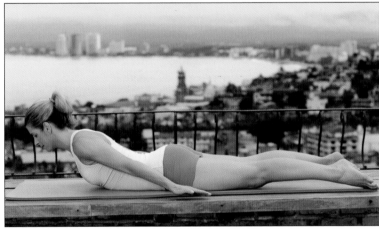

**POSITION 1:** Inhale to lift your shoulders to your ears and then back to slowly bring your chest off the mat. Slide your shoulders away from your ears as you lengthen your fingertips behind you, engaging your mid-back muscles. Exhale to lower your body and arms to the floor. Do 5 reps.

## FABULOUS FORM TIPS

○ Don't move your pelvis. Instead, make your hipbones and pubic bone flush with the mat.

○ Don't work with your shoulders anywhere near your ears. Imagine squeezing a couple of pencils under your armpits to engage your upper back muscles.

## the payoff:

Strengthens your posture muscles

# **1** single-leg hip extension

**sets -n- reps:** Do three sets of 5 reps.
**must-haves:** Nothing

○○○○

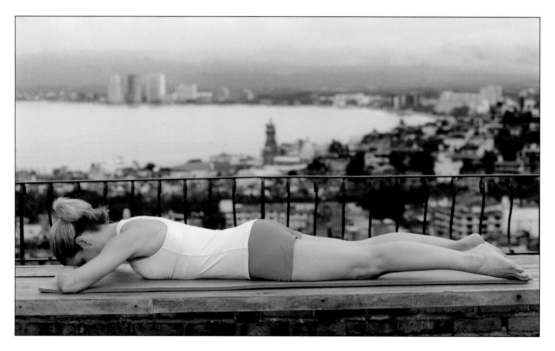

**STARTING POSITION:** Lie on your stomach with your legs straight and place your arms under your head, crossing them at your wrists, palms down. Rest your forehead on your hands and relax your upper back.

## **the payoff:**

Creates a strong and healthy lower back

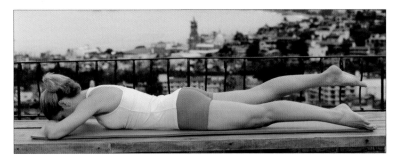

**POSITION 1:** Inhale to lift your right leg not too high off the mat. Pay attention to your pelvis—absolutely no movement! Hold for 3 to 5 seconds, and then lower your leg.

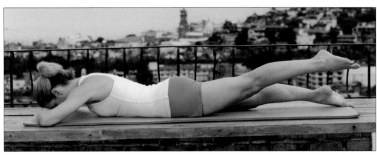

**POSITION 2:** Inhale to lift your left leg not too high off the mat. Again, maintain your stable (neutral) pelvis position. Hold for 3 to 5 seconds, and then lower your leg. Do 5 reps.

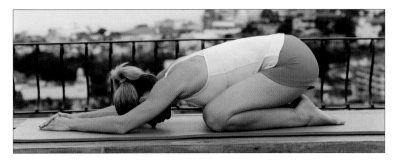

**POSITION 3:** Then move your hips to your heels and rest in what is called Child's Pose.

## FABULOUS FORM TIPS

- ❍ Practice good form to protect your lower back. Lift your belly button to your spine and firm up your fanny and hams. (You get a little extra booty work, too!)

- ❍ Maintain a neutral pelvis, with no pelvic tilt. (If you don't know what a pelvic tilt looks like, turn to page 11.)

- ❍ Don't put any pressure on your lower back. Immediately stop if you feel any lower back pain.

- ❍ Relax your upper back. Putting your shoulders by your ears is a no-no.

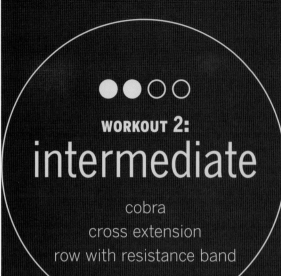

●●○○

**WORKOUT 2:**
# intermediate

cobra
cross extension
row with resistance band

---

**THE PAYOFF:**
## Lengthens your look!
## (Wouldn't you want that?)

---

**TOTAL TIME:** 15 to 20 minutes

**HOW OFTEN:** Spend two to four weeks building overall strength in your back. Now, focus on the micro-movements and really feeling this work in your midback—or that bra-line area. Remember, there should be no pain, pressure, or strain in your lower back. Do this workout three times a week on nonconsecutive days.

★ **PERFECT YOUR POSTURE,**
on page 202, offers more advice for
maximizing this workout.

**2 cobra**
○○○○

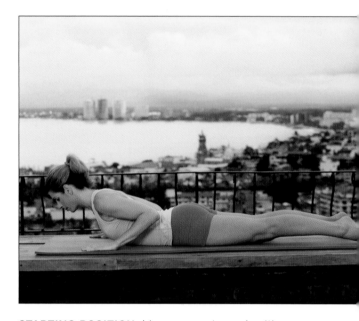

**STARTING POSITION:** Lie on your stomach with your legs straight and slightly open. Place the palms of your hands next to your shoulders on the floor.

## the payoff:
Creates a strong and healthy lower back

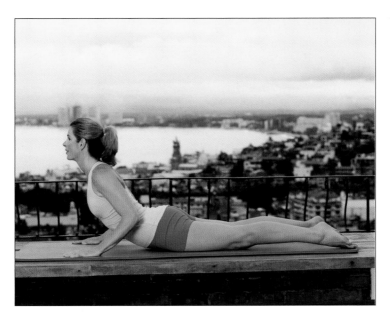

**POSITION 1:** Inhale to lift your chest off the mat. Important: Glue your arms to your ribs to help keep your shoulders from lifting to your ears. Do 5 to 8 reps.

# FABULOUS FORM TIPS

- ○ Don't lift your shoulders to your ears. Instead, glue your elbows to your ribs, which will prevent you from splaying out your arms to the sides.

- ○ Don't overarch your neck; your head should follow the alignment of your spine.

- ○ Don't push into your lower back. Instead, only come up to the point of no pressure in your lower back.

- ○ Open your chest by un-rounding your shoulders!

# **2** cross extension

**sets -n- reps:** Do three sets 5 to 8 reps.
**must-haves:** Nothing

○○○○

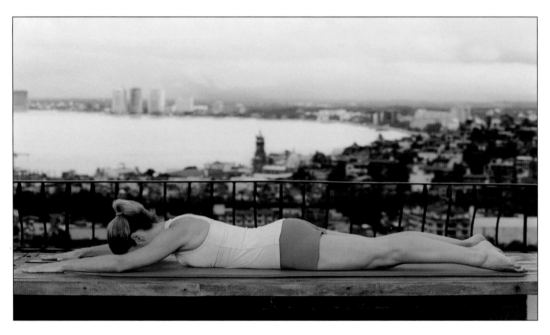

**STARTING POSITION:** Lie on your stomach with your legs straight and lengthen your arms over your head, palms down.

## **the payoff:**

Builds balance and strength between upper and lower back muscles!

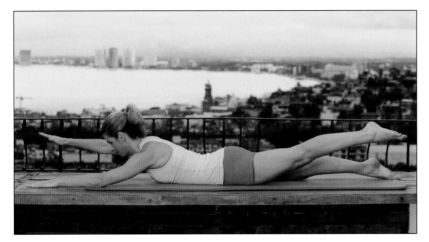

**POSITION 1:** Inhale to lift your right arm and left leg, keeping your hipbones down on the mat. Pay attention to your pelvis—absolutely no movement! Lower your arm and leg to the mat. Hold for 3 to 5 seconds, then switch sides.

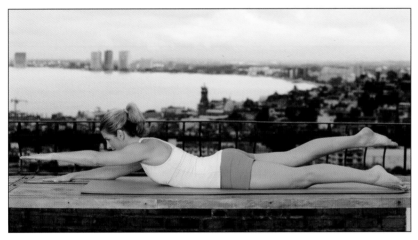

**POSITION 2:** Inhale to lift your left arm and right leg, keeping your hipbones down on the mat. Again, your pelvis shouldn't be moving. Hold for 3 to 5 seconds, then switch sides. Do 5 to 8 reps, and then rest in Child's Pose.

## FABULOUS FORM TIPS

○ Don't lift your shoulders to your ears, which is really hard not to do. Instead, lift from your bra-line area, making your midback work.

○ Practice good form to protect your lower back. Lift your belly button to your spine and firm up your fanny and hams. (You get a little extra booty work, too.)

○ Maintain a neutral pelvis, with no pelvic tilt. (If you don't know what a pelvic tilt looks like, turn to page 11.)

○ Look down and keep your head in line with your spine.

○ Lift from your midback. Imagine cracking a walnut between your shoulder blades.

# **2** row with resistance band

○○○○

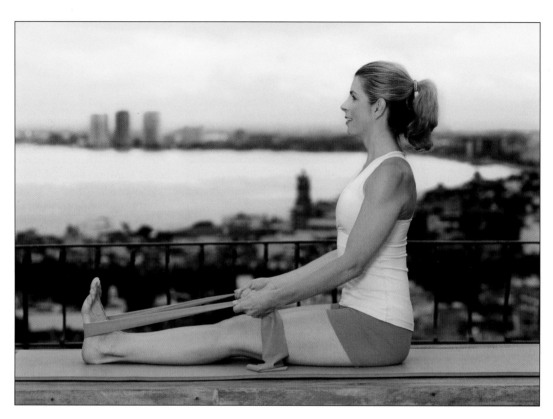

**STARTING POSITION:** Sit on your bottom with your legs straight or slightly bent and wrap a resistance band around your feet. Sit tall while holding the band in each hand, palms up.

## **the payoff:**

Lengthens your look and strengthens your lats

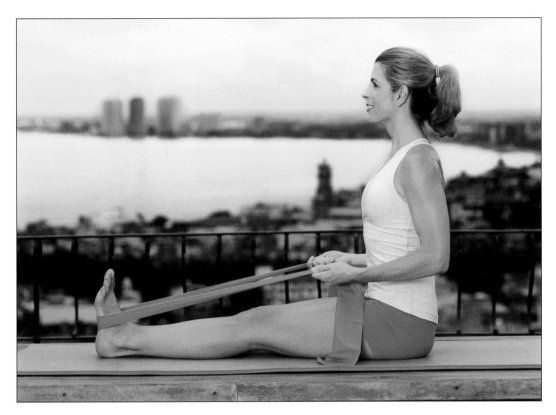

**POSITION 1:** Bend your elbows to slide your arms to the outside of your chest. Pause and return to the starting position. Do 12 to 15 reps.

## FABULOUS FORM TIPS

○ Don't swing your arms. Move with control as your knuckles face down.

○ Sit tall and follow all the good posture tips such as un-rounding your shoulders. Imagine cracking a walnut between your shoulder blades.

●●●○

**WORKOUT 3:**

# advanced

snorkel
snorkel with goalpost arms
lift and rotate (extension)

**THE PAYOFF:**
## Perfects your posture, hot stuff!

**TOTAL TIME:** 15 to 20 minutes

**HOW OFTEN:** Spend two to four weeks perfecting your posture. By now, you should be feeling this work in your midback; keep going! To up the workload, do these exercises on a bench or step. But if you don't have one or you feel this in your lower back, take the work to the mat. Do this workout three times a week on nonconsecutive days.

★ **PERFECT YOUR POSTURE,**
on page 202, offers more advice for
maximizing this workout.

# 3  snorkel

○○○○

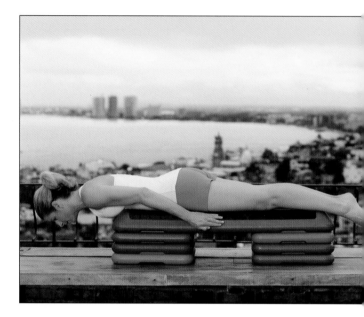

**STARTING POSITION:** Lie on your stomach with your chest off a bench or step and open your legs about shoulder-width apart. Straighten your arms by your sides, palms down.

## the payoff:

Straightens and strengthens
your back

**sets -n- reps:**   Do three sets of 8 to 10 reps.

**must-haves:**   Step with risers or bench

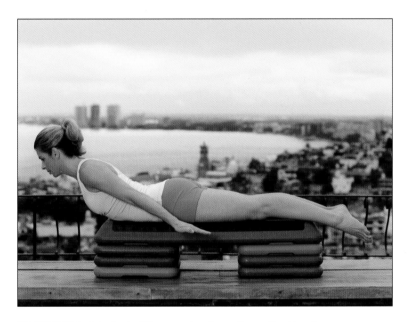

**POSITION 1:** Inhale to lift your chest up. Pay attention to your pelvis—absolutely no movement! Do 8 to 10 reps, then rest in Child's Pose.

# FABULOUS FORM TIPS

❍ Practice good form, especially because the workload for your lower back is harder. Lift your belly button to your spine and firm up your fanny and hams. (You get a little extra booty work, too.)

❍ Maintain a neutral pelvis, with no pelvic tilt. (If you don't know what a pelvic tilt looks like, turn to page 11.)

❍ There shouldn't be any pressure or pain in your lower back—ever.

❍ Un-round your shoulders as you lift into extension and then squeeze you midback to hold the exercise.

❍ Look at the floor so you don't strain your delicate neck muscles.

# **3** snorkel with goalpost arms

○ ○ ○ ○

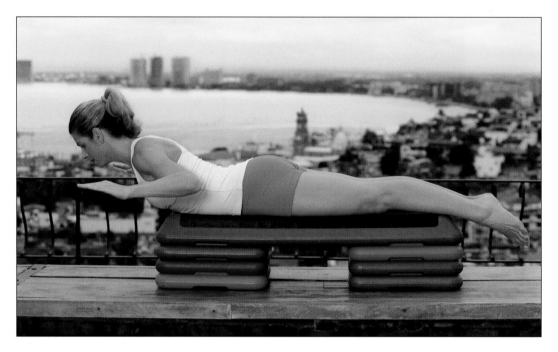

**STARTING POSITION:** Lie on your stomach with your chest off a bench or step and open your legs shoulder-width apart. This time, inhale to lift into an extension and hold. It's your midback muscles that are working hard to stabilize you. Move your arms so they are parallel to the floor as in a goal-post position. You should be able to see your fingers out to your sides, palms down.

## **the payoff:**

Strengthens your upper back-n-perfects your posture

**sets -n- reps:** Do three sets of 8 to 10 reps.

**must-haves:** Step with risers or bench

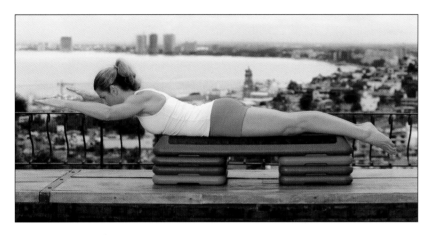

**POSITION 1:** Inhale to straighten your arms (not totally straight) in front of you.

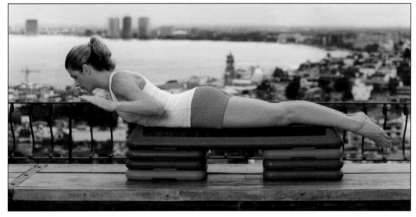

**POSITION 2:** Exhale to bring your arms back. Keep your chest lifted the whole time while doing the arm movements. Remember, there should be no strain, pain, or pressure in your lower back! Do 8 to 10 reps, then rest in Child's Pose.

# FABULOUS FORM TIPS

- ❍ Feel this work all over, especially on your side back muscles, or lats.

- ❍ Practice good form, especially because, wow, that's tons of work for your entire back! Lift your belly button to your spine and firm up your fanny and hams.

- ❍ Maintain a neutral pelvis and avoid a pelvic tilt. (If you don't know what a pelvic tilt looks like, turn to page 11.)

- ❍ There should be no pressure or pain in your lower back—ever.

- ❍ Don't worry about straightening your arms all the way. The focus is on bringing your arms back to engage your lats.

# **3** lift and rotate (extension)

○○○○

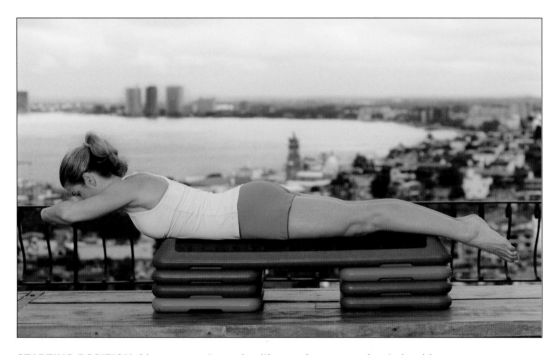

**STARTING POSITION:** Lie on your stomach with your legs open about shoulder-width apart. Move your arms in front of your forehead and cross your wrists so your elbows are out to your sides, palms down. Inhale to lift your chest off the mat and hold it by engaging your midback muscles.

## **the payoff:**

Bye-bye back fat—hello perfect posture!

**sets -n- reps:**    Do three sets of 8 to 10 reps.

**must-haves:**      Step with risers or bench

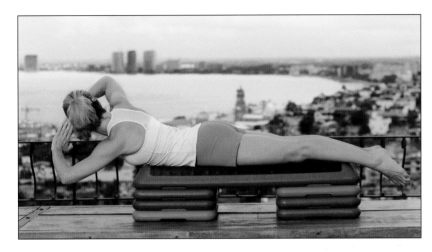

**POSITION 1:** Exhale to twist to the right, leading with your midback. You should be able to see your right elbow out of the corner of your eye.

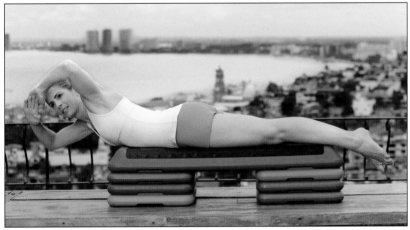

**POSITION 2:** Inhale to the starting position, then exhale and twist left, moving from your midback. Do 8 to 10 reps, then rest in Child's Pose.

# FABULOUS FORM TIPS

❍ Don't lift your shoulders to your ears; imagine cracking that walnut and moving from your midback to stabilize your shoulders.

❍ Practice good form, especially because this exercise is hard and takes concentration as you twist. Lift your belly button to your spine and firm up your fanny and hams.

❍ Maintain a neutral pelvis; avoid a pelvic tilt. (If you don't know what a pelvic tilt looks like, turn to page 11.)

❍ There should be no pain, strain, or pressure in your lower back—ever.

❍ Look at your elbow as you twist to keep your head aligned.

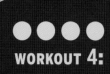

## WORKOUT 4:
# super advanced

snorkel with big ball
lift and rotate with big ball
single-leg bent-over row

---

### THE PAYOFF:
## Beats the back fat!

---

**TOTAL TIME:** 15 to 20 minutes

**HOW OFTEN:** Spend two to four weeks maintaining your posture and keeping your back healthy and strong. The exercises here are super hard, so drape over the ball anytime you need to stretch your lower back. Remember, there should be no pain, strain, or pressure in your lower back—ever. Do this workout three times a week on nonconsecutive days.

★ **PERFECT YOUR POSTURE,**
on page 202, offers more advice for
maximizing this workout.

# 4  snorkel with
○○○○

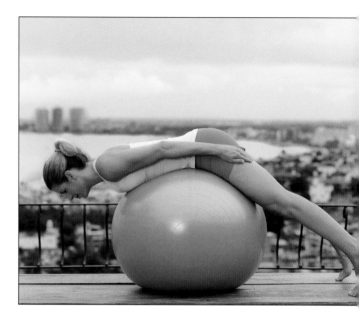

**STARTING POSITION:** Lie on your stomach on the ball with your legs straight and open about shoulder-width apart. Round your belly over the ball and place your hands on the back of your legs, palms down.

## the payoff:
Builds posture strength and beats the back fat.

# big ball

**sets -n- reps:** Do three sets of 8 to 10 reps.
**must-haves:** Stability ball

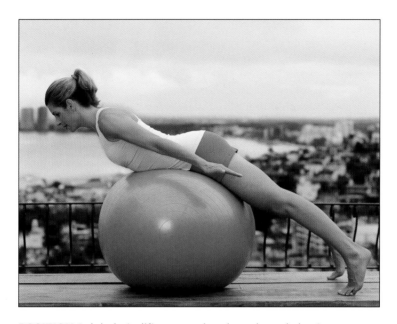

**POSITION 1:** Inhale to lift up your head, neck, and chest. Pay attention to your pelvis. There should be absolutely no movement! Do 8 to 10 reps, then drape over the ball if you need a rest.

## FABULOUS FORM TIPS

❍ Move from your midback. Focus on the contraction to get the most out of this work.

❍ Look in front of you so as not to strain your delicate neck muscles.

❍ Don't lift your shoulders to your ears. Imagine cracking that walnut, moving from your midback to stabilize your shoulders.

❍ Practice good form because the ball challenges your stability, making your lower back work that much harder. Lift your belly button to your spine and firm up your fanny and hams.

❍ Maintain a neutral pelvis, with no pelvic tilt. (If you don't know what a pelvic tilt looks like, turn to page 11.)

❍ There should be no pain, strain, or pressure in your lower back—ever.

# **4** lift and rotate with big ball

○○○○

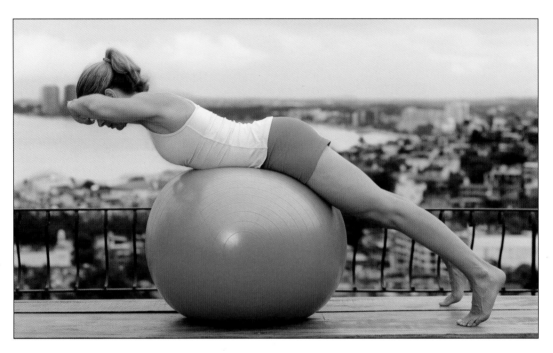

**STARTING POSITION:** Lie on your stomach on the ball with your legs straight and open about shoulder-width apart. Move your arms in front of your forehead and overlap your fingers so your elbows are out to your sides, palms down. Inhale to lift your chest up.

## **the payoff:**
Delivers such a beautiful strong back

**sets -n- reps:** Do three sets of 8 to 10 reps.
**must-haves:** Stability ball

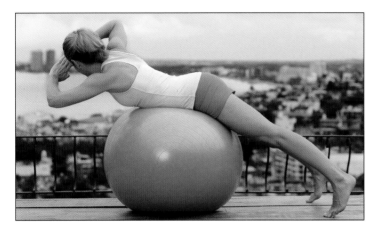

**POSITION 1:** Exhale to twist right, moving from your upper back.

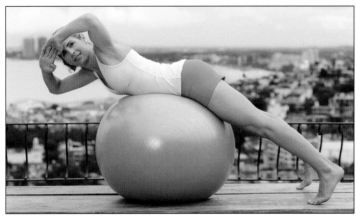

**POSITION 2:** Inhale to the starting position and then exhale to twist left, moving from your upper back. Do 8 to 10 reps, and then drape over the ball to rest your back.

# FABULOUS FORM TIPS

○ Move from you midback. It's your midback that stabilizes you and works hard while you're on the ball.

○ Look at your elbow to follow the alignment of your spine and to avoid straining your delicate neck muscles.

○ Don't lift your shoulders to your ears. Imagine cracking that walnut, moving from your midback to stabilize your shoulders.

○ Practice good form because the ball challenges your stability, making the workload harder on your lower back. Lift your belly button to your spine and firm up your fanny and hams.

○ Maintain a neutral pelvis, with no pelvic tilt. (If you don't know what a pelvic tilt looks like, turn to page 11.)

○ There should be no pain, strain, or pressure in your lower back—ever.

# **4** single-leg bent-over row

○○○○

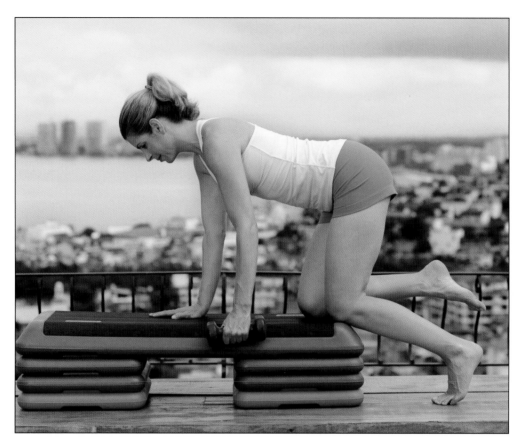

**STARTING POSITION:** Kneel on your step in a comfortable position. Hold a 5- to 10-pound (2- to 4.5-kg) dumbbell in your left hand and bend from your waist. Straighten your left arm, palms facing in, and rest your right hand on the step for stability.

## **the payoff:**
Works your lats luscious!

**sets -n- reps:** Do three sets of 10 reps.

**must-haves:** A pair of 5- to 10-pound (2- to 4.5-kg) dumbbells, and a step with risers or bench

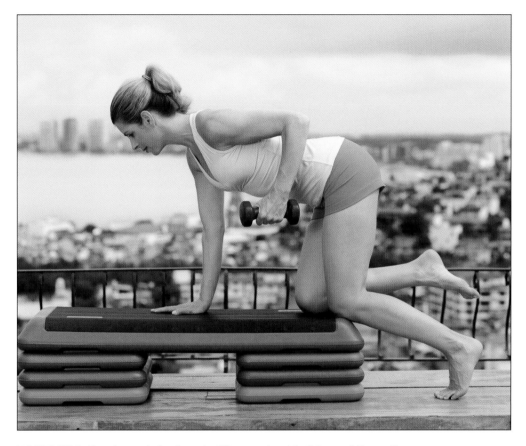

**POSITION 1:** Bend your left elbow to lift your dumbbell toward the ceiling. The dumbbell will slide on the outside of your chest. Pause and return to the starting position. Do 10 reps, then switch arms and do another 10 reps.

## FABULOUS FORM TIPS

○ Don't move your pelvis. Use your abs to stabilize you and keep your hipbones facing down.

○ Don't swing your arms. Move with control as your knuckles face out and your elbows are in line with your shoulders.

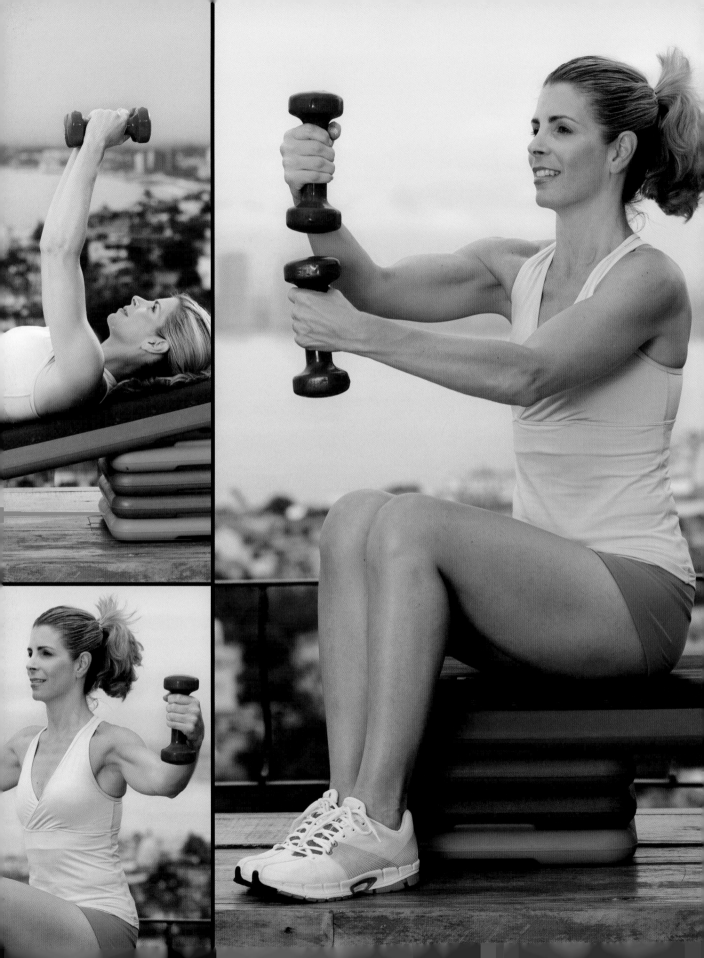

# chapter 9

# THE DEEP PLUNGE

| | the payoff | total time | how often | sets -n- reps | must-haves |
|---|---|---|---|---|---|
| **WORKOUT 1:**<br>**beginner**<br>○○○○<br><br>Chest Press<br>Push-up on Your Knees<br>Chest Fly (Alternating Arms) | Sculpts your chest stunning! | 15 to 20 minutes | Do this workout 3 times a week on non-consecutive days, such as Mon., Wed., and Fri. | Do three sets of 10 to 12 reps. | Pair of 5- to 10-pound (2- to 4.5-kg) dumbbells and a step or bench |
| **WORKOUT 2:**<br>**intermediate**<br>○○○○<br><br>Push-up with a Twist (knees)<br>Chest Fly<br>Push-up | Sexifies your chest! | 15 to 20 minutes | Do this workout 3 times a week on non-consecutive days, such as Mon., Wed., and Fri. | Do three sets of 12 to 15 reps. | Pair of 5- to 10-pound (2- to 4.5-kg) dumbbells and a bench or step |
| **WORKOUT 3–4:**<br>**advanced to super advanced**<br>○○○○<br>○○○○<br><br>Push-up with a Twist<br>One-Arm Chest Fly on Ball<br>Decline Push-up | Gives you such a lovely lift—and delectable décolletage! | 15 to 20 minutes | Do this workout 3 times a week on non-consecutive days, such as Mon., Wed., and Fri. | Do three sets of 15 to 20 reps. | Pair of 5- to 10-pound (2- to 4.5-kg) dumbbells, stability ball, and a step or bench |

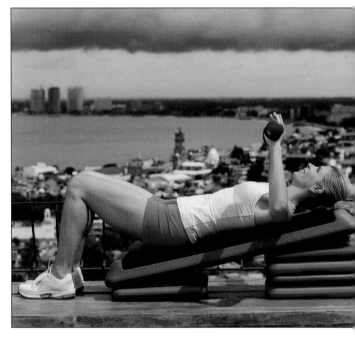

**STARTING POSITION:** Using 5- to 10-pound (2- to 4.5-kg) dumbbells, lie flat on your back, either on an inclined bench or step. Lower your arms out to the sides so your elbows are in line with shoulders. You might see the weights in your peripheral vision.

## the payoff:
The strongest and sexiest chest you can imagine!

---

●○○○

**WORKOUT 1:**
# beginner
chest press
push-up on your knees
chest fly (alternating arms)

---

**THE PAYOFF:**
## Sculpts your chest stunning!

---

**TOTAL TIME:** 15 to 20 minutes

**HOW OFTEN:** Spend two to four weeks building overall strength in your chest. The form is basically the same from exercise to exercise, but do practice! Do this workout three times a week on nonconsecutive days.

★ **GET A NATURAL LIFT,**
on page 203, offers more advice for
maximizing this workout.

**sets -n- reps:** Do three sets of 10 to 12 reps.

**must-haves:** Pair of 5- to 10-pound (2- to 4.5-kg) dumbbells and a step or bench

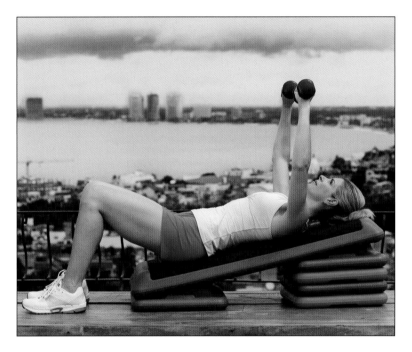

**POSITION 1:** Raise your arms up and together, until the dumbbells almost touch. Pause, and then slowly lower your arms. Do 10 to 12 reps.

# FABULOUS FORM TIPS

○ Don't swing your arms. Use control to lift and lower your weights.

○ Don't lift your lower back off the bench. If you can't do the exercise without your back lifting off the bench, engage your abs to support your lower back. Next, drop down in weight. Your weights may be too heavy if you can't stabilize your torso.

○ Focus on squeezing and lifting. You may feel a slight stretch across your chest in the starting position.

# 1 push-up on your knees

**sets -n- reps:** Do three sets of 10 to 12 reps.
**must-haves:** Nothing

○○○○

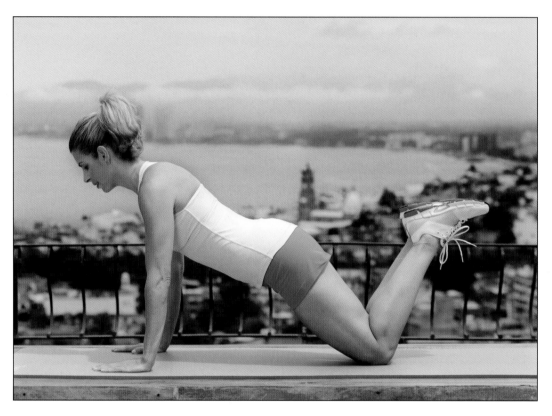

**STARTING POSITION:** While on your knees, place your hands on the floor directly under your shoulders, palms down.

## the payoff:

Strengthens your chest muscles!

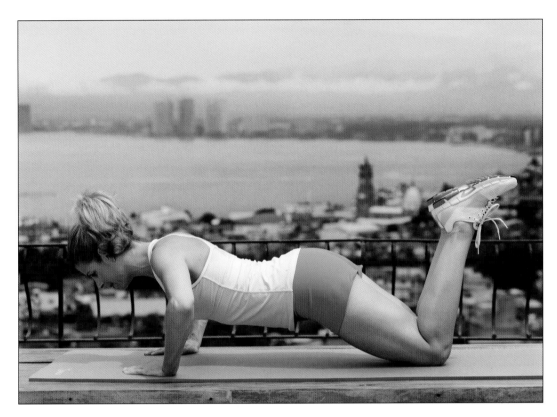

**POSITION 1:** Bend your elbows out to the sides and lower your body to the floor. Push up to the starting position. Do 10 to 12 reps.

## FABULOUS FORM TIPS

❍ Don't let your belly sag. Gently lift your belly button to your spine to strengthen your tummy while supporting your lower back.

❍ Don't elevate your shoulders. Drop your shoulders away from your ears to engage your upper back.

❍ Don't drop your head. Look at the floor as you lengthen from the top of your head.

❍ Don't overdo the push-up. For example, only lower down so your shoulders are in line with your elbows. Don't go any lower or you may put too much pressure on your elbow joints, and your chest doesn't get to work as hard.

# 1 chest fly (alternating arms)

○○○○

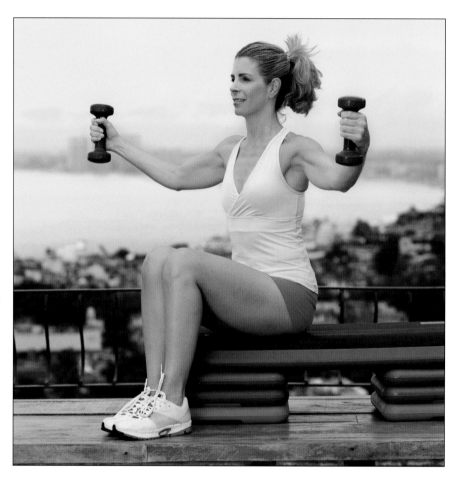

**STARTING POSITION:** Using 5- to 10-pound (2- to 4.5-kg) dumbbells, sit on either a bench or a step. Open your arms out to your sides so your palms face each other.

## the payoff:

Tones and tightens upper arms and chest

**sets -n- reps:** Do three sets of 10 to 12 reps.

**must-haves:** Pair of 5- to 10-pound (2- to 4.5-kg) dumbbells and a step or bench

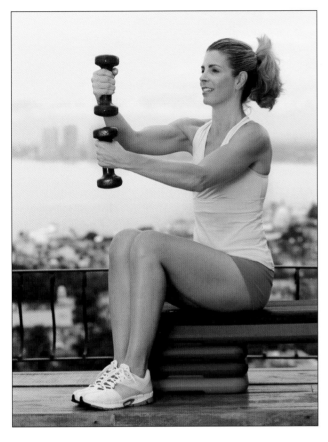

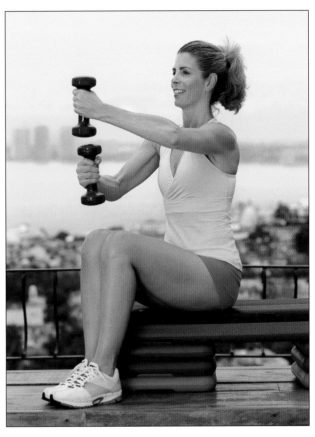

**POSITION 1:** Bring your arms together so your right hand is on top of your left hand.

**POSITION 2:** Open your arms and then bring your arms together so your left hand is on top of your right hand. Complete both sides to make one rep and do 10 to 12 reps.

## FABULOUS FORM TIPS

- ❍ Don't swing your arms. Instead, use controlled movements.

- ❍ Engage your abs so you can sit tall.

- ❍ Make an arc-shaped movement with your arms. Imagine hugging a huge tree.

- ❍ Squeeze your chest before moving your arms.

## WORKOUT 2:
# intermediate

push-up with a twist
chest fly
push-up

---

**THE PAYOFF:**
## Sexifies your chest!

**TOTAL TIME:** 15 to 20 minutes

**HOW OFTEN:** Spend two to four weeks developing a stunning, strong chest. Do this workout three times a week on nonconsecutive days.

★ **GET A NATURAL LIFT,** on page 203, offers more advice for maximizing this workout.

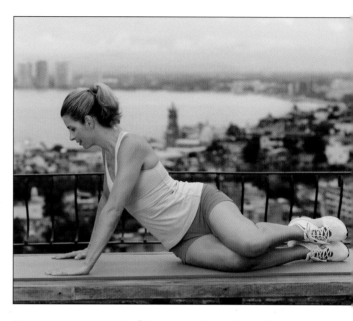

**STARTING POSITION:** Sit on your right hip and stack your knees. Twist your torso to the right to place your hands on the floor about shoulder-width apart, palms down.

## the payoff:
A chest that's the best

# twist (knees)

**sets -n- reps:** Do three sets of 12 to 15 reps.
**must-haves:** Nothing

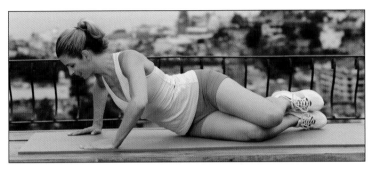

**POSITION 1:** Bend your elbows out to the sides to lower your body and then push up. You should feel this work all down your right side—chest, arm, and waist. Do 12 to 15 reps, and then switch sides.

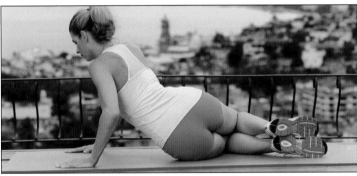

**POSITION 2:** Sit on your left hip and stack your knees. Twist your torso to the left to place your hands on the floor about shoulder-width apart, palms down.

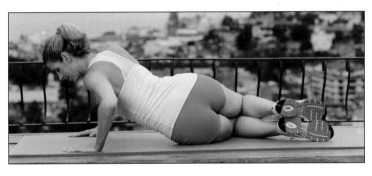

**POSITION 3:** Bend your elbows out to the sides to lower your body and then push up. You should feel this work all down your left side—chest, arm, and waist. Do 12 to 15 reps, and then switch sides.

## FABULOUS FORM TIPS

○ Don't let your belly sag. Instead, gently lift your belly button to your spine to strengthen your abs and give your lower back support.

○ Don't elevate your shoulders. Draw them away from your ears.

○ Don't drop your head. Look at the floor as you lengthen from the top of your head.

○ Twist from your mid-back or last rib to get lots of waist work.

# **2** chest fly

○○○○

| | |
|---|---|
| **sets -n- reps:** | Do three sets of 12 to 15 reps. |
| **must-haves:** | Pair of 5- to 10-pound (2- to 4.5-kg) dumbbells and a bench or step |

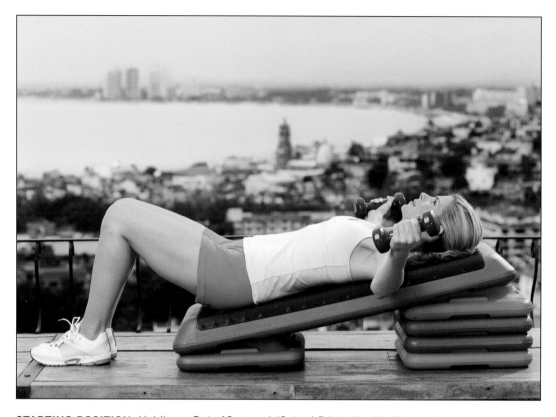

**STARTING POSITION:** Holding a 5- to 10-pound (2- to 4.5-kg) dumbbell in each hand, lie flat on your back, either on an inclined bench or a step. Open your arms out to your side so your forearms face up, palms up.

## the payoff:

Develops a strong and sexy chest

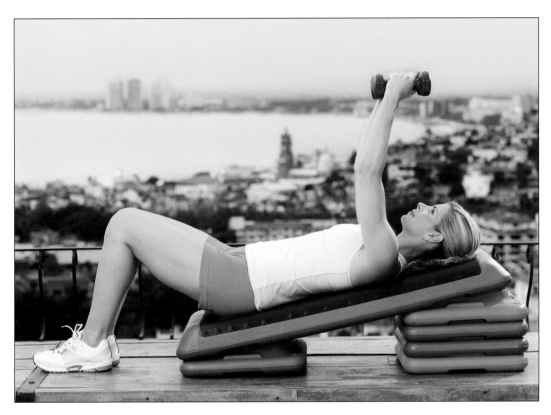

**POSITION 1:** Raise your arms up and together. Pause, and then slowly lower your arms. Do 12 to 15 reps.

## FABULOUS FORM TIPS

- ❍ Don't swing your arms. Use controlled movements to lift and lower your weights.

- ❍ Don't lift your lower back off the bench. Engage your abs to support your lower back. You may have to drop down in dumbbell weight if they are too heavy so that you can stabilize your torso.

- ❍ Make an arc-shaped movement with your arms. Imagine hugging a huge tree.

- ❍ Contract your chest before you move your arms.

# 2 push-up

○○○○

| | |
|---|---|
| **sets -n- reps:** | Do three sets of 12 to 15 reps. |
| **must-haves:** | Nothing |

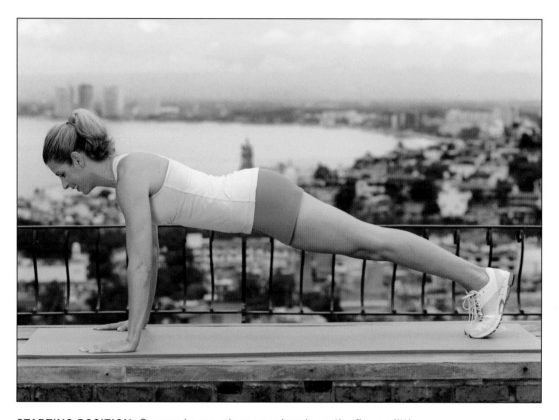

**STARTING POSITION:** On your knees, place your hands on the floor a little wider than shoulder-width, palms down. With your toes curled under, place your heels together and lift your legs, pelvis, and torso off the floor in one motion.

## the payoff:

Strengthens–oh-so-strong (real women do pushups)

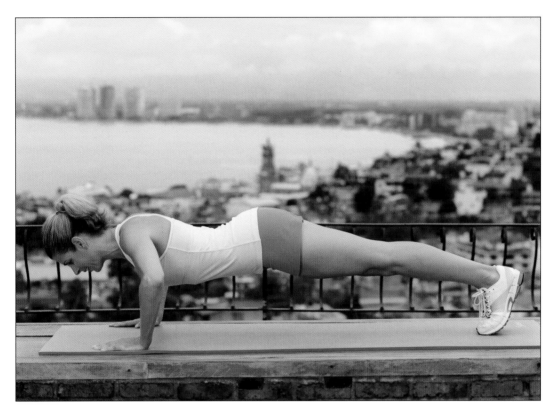

**POSITION 1:** Bend your elbows out to the sides to lower your body to the floor. Push up to a plank position. Do 12 to 15 reps.

## FABULOUS FORM TIPS

○ Don't let your belly sag. Gently lift your belly button to your spine to strengthen your abs and support your lower back.

○ Don't forget to firm up your fanny, inner thighs, and pelvic floor. Oh-so-much power is wasted if you don't use 'em!

○ Don't elevate your shoulders. Instead, draw them away from your ears.

○ Don't drop your head. Look at the floor as you lengthen from the top of your head.

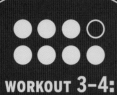

## WORKOUT 3–4:

# advanced to super advanced

push-up with a twist
one-arm chest fly on ball
decline push-up

---

**THE PAYOFF:**

## Gives you such a lovely lift— and delectable décolletage!

---

**TOTAL TIME:** 15 to 20 minutes

**HOW OFTEN:** You're on your way. Skimpy camisoles and sexy tank tops will both look dazzling! The ball ups the challenge, so focus on your chest and then some! Do this workout three times a week on nonconsecutive days.

★ **GET A NATURAL LIFT,**
on page 203, offers more advice for
maximizing this workout.

# push-up with a

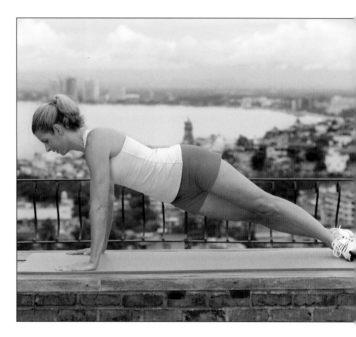

**STARTING POSITION:** Sit on your right hip and stack your knees. Twist your torso to the right and place your hands on the floor a little wider than shoulder-width apart, palms down. Straighten your legs so the right leg is underneath, squeezing your legs together to support your torso.

## the payoff:

An über-amazing upper body

# twist

**sets -n- reps:** Do three sets of 15 to 20 reps.
**must-haves:** Nothing

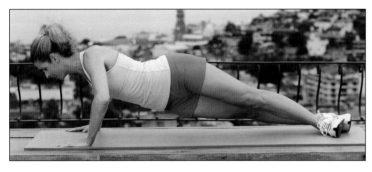

**POSITION 1:** Bend your elbows out to the sides to lower your body, and then push up. You should really feel this work down the entire right side of your chest, arm, and waist. Do 15 to 20 reps, then switch sides.

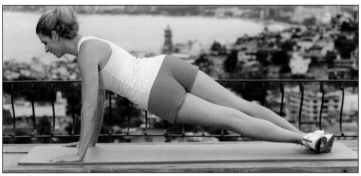

**POSITION 2:** Sit on your left hip and stack your knees. Twist your torso to the left and place your hands on the floor a little wider than shoulder-width apart, palms down. Straighten your legs so the left leg is underneath, squeezing your legs together to support your torso.

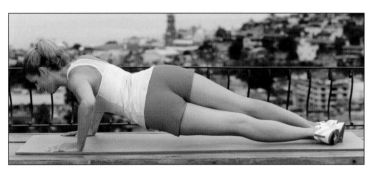

**POSITION 3:** Bend your elbows out to the sides to lower your body, and then push up. You should really feel this work down the entire left side of your chest, arm, and waist. Do 15 to 20 reps, then switch sides.

## FABULOUS FORM TIPS

○ Don't let your waist sag. Gently lift your hips to the sky to get the delicious waist work and provide lower back support.

○ Squeeze your legs together to give you a little extra power when doing the push-up.

○ Don't lift your shoulders. Draw them down to engage your upper back muscles.

○ Don't drop your head. Look at the floor as you lengthen from the top of your head.

# 3-4 one-arm chest fly on ball

○○○○
○○○○

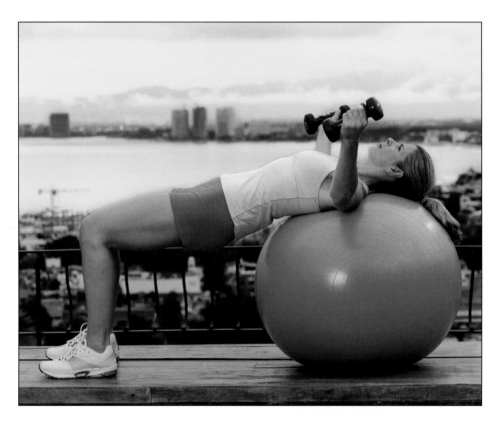

**STARTING POSITION:** Holding a 5- to 10-pound (2- to 4.5-kg) dumbbell in each hand, sit on the ball. Walk your legs out from the ball until your upper back and neck are on the ball, and then lift your hips to the ceiling so you're in a bridge position. When you're stable, open your arms out to your sides so your forearms face up, palms up.

## the payoff:

Gets your chest "cami-ready!"

**sets -n- reps:** Do three sets of 15 to 20 reps.

**must-haves:** Pair of 5- to 10-pound (2- to 4.5-kg) dumbbells and a stability ball

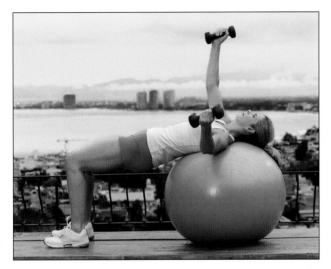

**POSITION 1:** Raise your right arm up, making a perfect arc with your arm. Pause, and then slowly lower your arm.

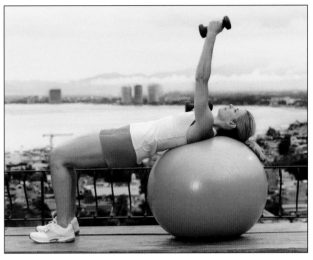

**POSITION 2:** Raise your left arm up, making a perfect arc with your arm. Pause, and then slowly lower your arm. Do 15 to 20 reps.

# FABULOUS FORM TIPS

- ❍ Don't swing your arms. Use controlled movements as you lift one arm at a time.

- ❍ Don't shift your hips as you lift your arm. Use your booty to help stabilize you in the bridge position.

- ❍ Make an arc-shaped movement with your arms. Imagine hugging a huge tree.

- ❍ Squeeze your chest before you move your arms.

# 3-4 decline push-up

○○○○
○○○○

**sets -n- reps:** Do three sets of 15 to 20 reps.
**must-haves:** A step or bench

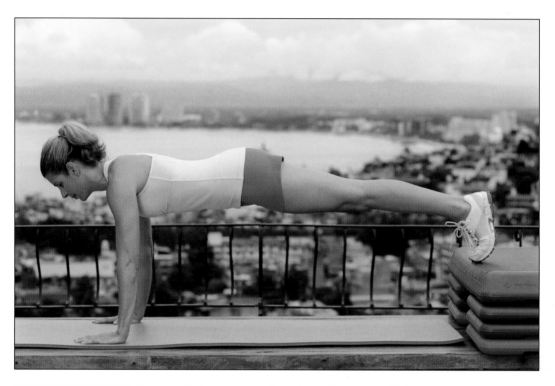

**STARTING POSITION:** Put your feet on a step, about four risers or so high, and place your hands on the floor directly under your shoulders, palms down. Lift your legs, pelvis, and torso off the floor into a plank position.

## the payoff:

Works your chest super-strong!

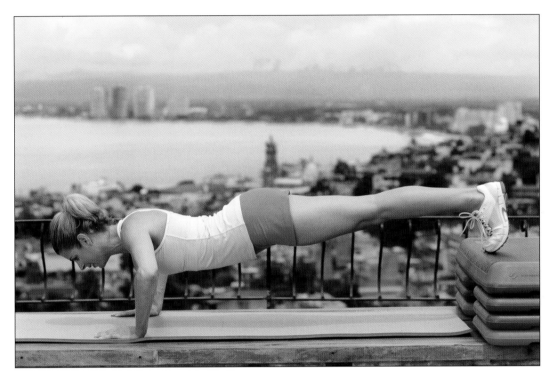

**POSITION 1:** Bend your elbows out to the sides and lower your body to the floor. Push up to a plank position. Do 15 to 20 reps.

## FABULOUS FORM TIPS

❍ Don't let your belly sag. Gently lift your belly button to your spine to strengthen your abs and support your lower back.

❍ Firm up your fanny, inner thighs, and pelvic floor. Oh-so-much power is wasted if you don't use them!

❍ Don't do this exercise if you have a shoulder injury. Doing a push-up on a decline puts extra work on your shoulders.

❍ Make sure your shoulders are away from your ears and engage the muscles of your upper back.

❍ Don't drop your head. Look at the floor as you lengthen from the top of your head.

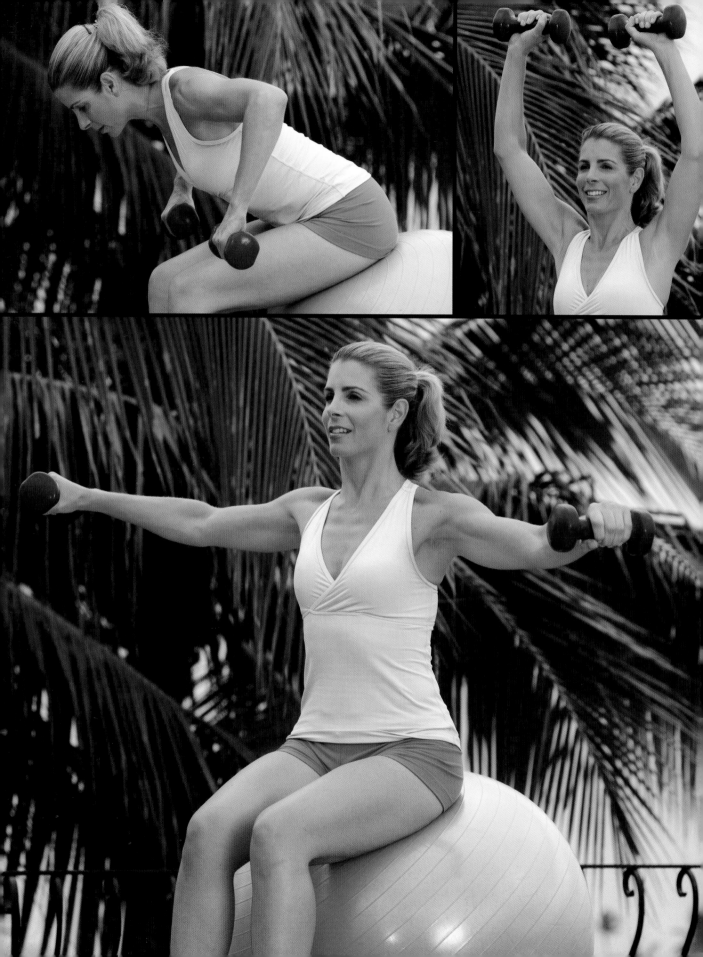

# chapter 10

# SCULPTED SEXY SHOULDERS

| | | the payoff | total time | how often | sets -n- reps | must-haves |
|---|---|---|---|---|---|---|
| **WORKOUT 1–2:**<br>beginner to intermediate<br><br>Shoulder Press<br>Side Raises<br>Bent-Arm Bent-Over Raise | ○○○○<br>○○○○ | Gives you balanced and beautiful shoulders! | 15 to 20 minutes | Do this workout 3 times a week on non-consecutive days, such as Mon., Wed., and Fri. | Do three sets of 10 to 12 reps. | Stability ball, step or bench, and pair of 5- to 10-pound (2- to 4.5-kg) dumbbells |
| **WORKOUT 3–4:**<br>advanced to super advanced<br><br>Front-Arm Raises<br>Side-Arm Raises<br>Reverse Fly | ○○○○<br>○○○○ | Gives your stunning and strong shoulders! | 15 to 20 minutes | Do this workout 3 times a week on non-consecutive days, such as Mon., Wed., and Fri. | Do three sets of 15 to 20 reps. | Pair of 5- to 10-pound (2- to 4.5-kg) dumbbells and stability ball (if you want) |

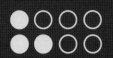

## WORKOUT 1–2:
# beginner to intermediate

shoulder press
side raises
bent-arm
bent-over raise

---

**THE PAYOFF:**
## Gives you balanced and beautiful shoulders!

---

**TOTAL TIME:** 15 to 20 minutes

**HOW OFTEN:** Spend two to four weeks developing overall strength in your shoulders to keep them strong for everyday life. Focus on good form to get strong, sexy shoulders and a sexy tummy. Do this workout three times a week on nonconsecutive days.

★ **SCULPTED SEXY SHOULDER TIPS,** on page 203, offers more advice for maximizing this workout.

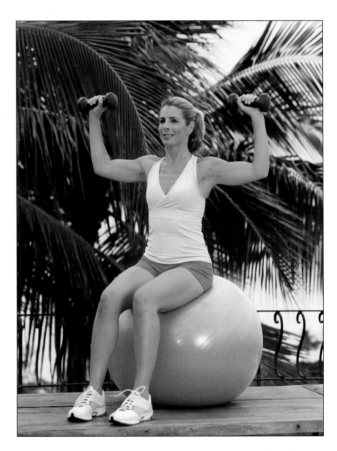

**STARTING POSITION:** Sit on a ball with your feet about hip-width apart. Hold a 5- to 10-pound (2- to 4.5-kg) dumbbell in each hand and bring your arms out to your sides in a goalpost position.

## the payoff:
Stunning shoulder definition

**sets -n- reps:** Do three sets of 10 to 12 reps.

**must-haves:** Stability ball and pair of 5- to 10-pound (2- to 4.5-kg) dumbbells

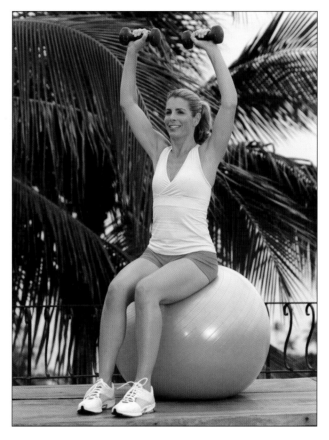

**POSITION 1:** Lift your arms up toward the ceiling in a smooth, controlled press and lower your arms. Do 10 to 12 reps.

# FABULOUS FORM TIPS

○ Don't lift your chest. Instead, focus on dropping your rib cage toward your hips, but keep your back straight.

○ Use slow and controlled movements to build overall strength in your shoulders—always!

○ Don't lock your elbows when straightening your arms because you'll take the work out of the shoulder muscle while putting needless pressure on your elbow joints.

# 1–2 side raises

○○○○
○○○○

**sets -n- reps:** Do three sets of 10 to 12 reps.

**must-haves:** Stability ball and pair of 5- to 10-pound (2- to 4.5-kg) dumbbells

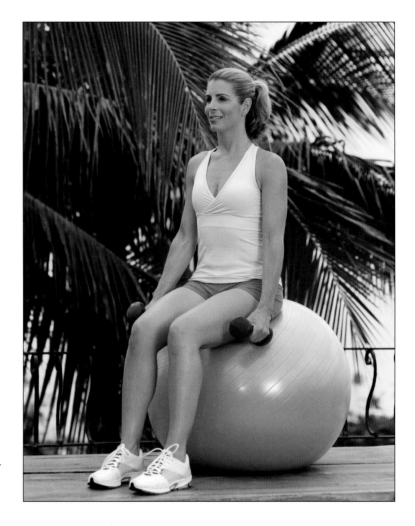

**STARTING POSITION:** Sit on a ball with your feet about hip-width apart. Hold a 5- to 10-pound (2- to 4.5-kg) dumbbell in each hand and lower your arms by your sides.

## the payoff:

Sculpts your mid shoulders-sexy!

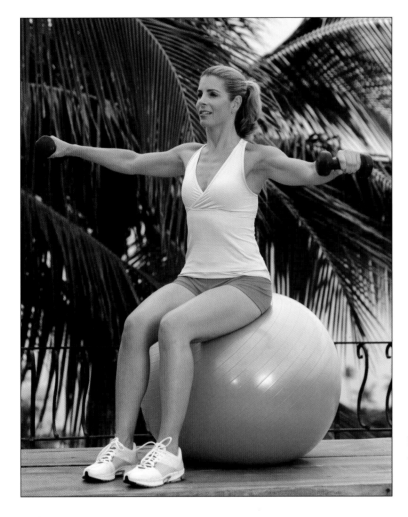

**POSITION 1:** Lift your arms up to the sides, shoulder height, in a smooth, controlled motion. Do 10 to 12 reps.

## FABULOUS FORM TIPS

- ❍ Don't lift your chest. Focus on dropping your rib cage toward your hips, but keep your back straight.

- ❍ Don't lift your arms higher than your shoulders, which ensures that you work the middle delt—always!

- ❍ Keep your arms straight to better isolate the middle delt.

# 1-2 bent-arm bent-over raise

○○○○
○○○○

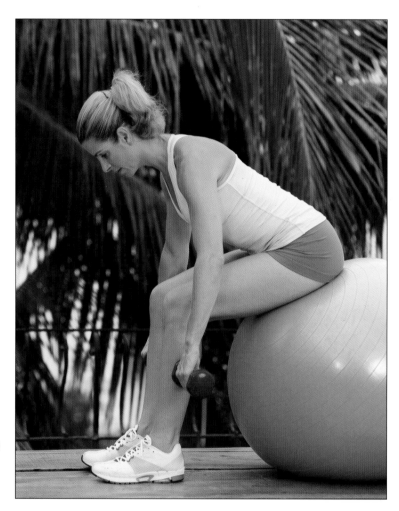

**STARTING POSITION:** Sit on a ball with your feet about hip-width apart. Hold a 5- to 10-pound (2- to 4.5-kg) dumbbell in each hand and bend over from the waist. Turn on your abs to support your lower back. Hang your arms in front, knuckles out, in line with your shoulders.

## the payoff:

Defines your back shoulders-lovely!

**sets -n- reps:**  Do three sets of 10 to 12 reps.

**must-haves:**  Stability ball and pair of 5- to 10-pound (2- to 4.5-kg) dumbbells

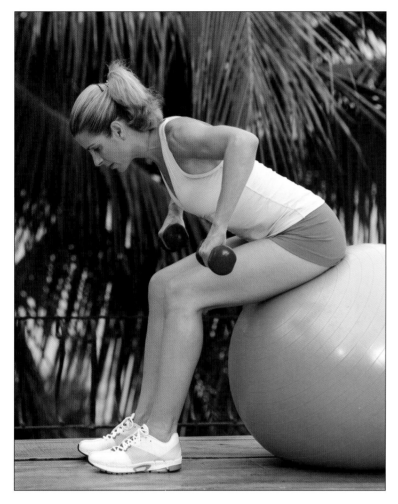

**POSITION 1:** Lift your arms up and out to the sides so your elbows point to the ceiling, making goalpost arms. Make sure you lift your arms only to shoulder height, bringing your shoulders blades together. Do 10 to 12 reps.

## FABULOUS FORM TIPS

○ Don't round your shoulders forward; keep your chest lifted and shoulders back.

○ Don't swing your arms. Move with control.

○ Don't lift your arms higher than your shoulders. Engage your upper back muscles to crack a walnut between your shoulder blades. Well, at least imagine it!

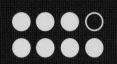

**WORKOUT 3-4:**

# advanced to super advanced

front-arm raises
side-arm raises
reverse fly

---

**THE PAYOFF:**
## Gives you stunning and strong shoulders!

---

**TOTAL TIME:** 15 to 20 minutes

**HOW OFTEN:** Spend two to four weeks to build strength and stability in your shoulders by including work for the deep stabilizing muscles or rotators. Don't lift weights that are too heavy; otherwise, momentum will kick in—and you don't want that! Do this workout three times a week on nonconsecutive days.

★ **SCULPTED SEXY SHOULDER TIPS,** on page 203, offers more advice for maximizing this workout.

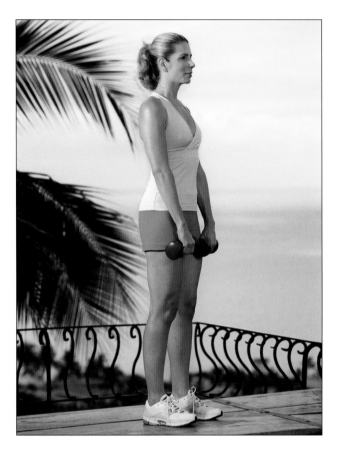

**STARTING POSITION:** Stand with your legs hip-width apart with soft knees. Hold a 5- to 10-pound (2- to 4.5-kg) dumbbell in each hand. Straighten your arms so the dumbbells touch the tops of your thighs, knuckles up.

## the payoff:

Rock-solid delts!

**sets -n- reps:** Do three sets of 15 to 20 reps.

**must-haves:** Pair of 5- to 10-pound (2- to 4.5-kg) dumbbells and stability ball (if you want)

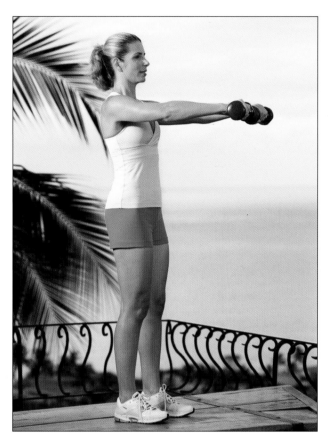

**POSITION 1:** Lift the dumbbells straight in front of you, about shoulder height. Pause slightly, and then return to the starting position. Do 15 to 20 reps.

## FABULOUS FORM TIPS

❍ Don't lift your shoulders to your ears. Use your shoulder muscles to lift your arms—not your delicate shoulder joints.

❍ Don't swing your arms. Momentum is a no-no when lifting your dumbbells because your shoulders tend to be overworked and prone to injury. Not to mention, if you're just swinging through the motion, you're not building strength.

❍ Slightly bend your elbows, keeping the focus on your front delt.

# 3-4 side-arm raises

○○○○
○○○○

| **sets -n- reps:** | Do three sets of 15 to 20 reps. |
|---|---|
| **must-haves:** | Pair of 5- to 10-pound (2- to 4.5-kg) dumbbells and stability ball (if you want) |

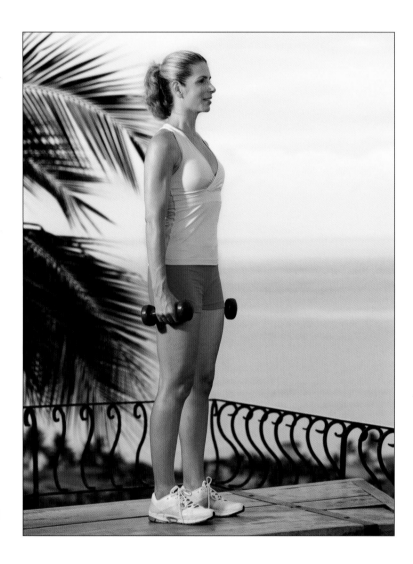

**STARTING POSITION:** Stand with your feet hip-width apart with soft knees. Hold a 5- to 10-pound (2- to 4.5-kg) dumbbell in each hand, knuckles up. Straighten your arms so the dumbbells touch the sides of your thighs, thumbs pointing in.

## the payoff:

Sculpts your mid-shoulders.

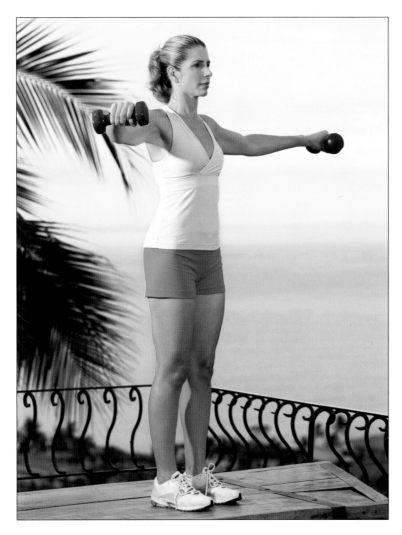

**POSITION 1:** With a slight bend in your elbows, lift your arms out to your sides so the dumbbells end up just about shoulder height. Pause, and then return to the starting position. Do 15 to 20 reps.

## FABULOUS FORM TIPS

❍ Don't bend your wrists. Maintain strong arms.

❍ Don't lift your shoulders to your ears. Use your shoulder muscles to lift your arms—not your delicate shoulder joints.

# 3-4 reverse fly

○○○○
○○○○

**sets -n- reps:** Do three sets of 15 to 20 reps.

**must-haves:** Pair of 5- to 10-pound (2- to 4.5-kg) dumbbells and stability ball (if you want)

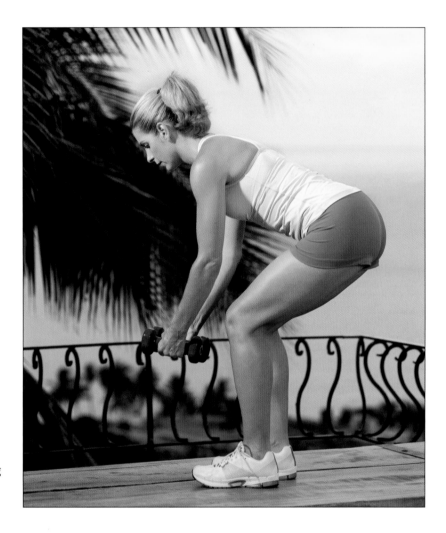

**STARTING POSITION:** Stand in a squat position with your feet about hip-width apart. Hold a 5- to 10-pound (2- to 4.5-kg) dumbbell in each hand and bend over from the waist. Turn on your abs to support your lower back. Hang your arms in front, knuckles out, in line with your shoulders.

## the payoff:

Strengthens your back delts and defines your posture!

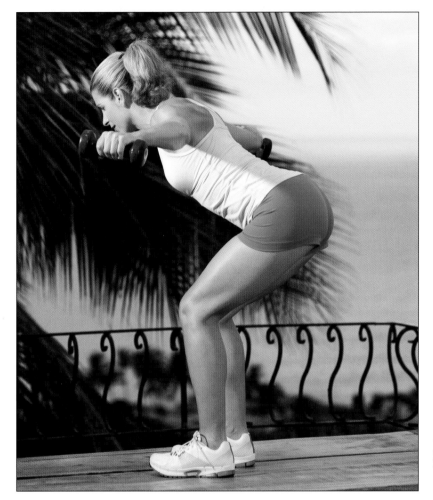

**POSITION 1:** Lift your arms up and out to the sides until your arms are parallel with the floor, about shoulder height, bringing your shoulders blades together. Your elbows should be slightly bent. Do 15 to 20 reps.

## FABULOUS FORM TIPS

○ Don't round your shoulders forward. Keep your chest lifted and your shoulders back.

○ Don't lift your arms higher than your shoulders. Engage your upper back muscles to crack a walnut between your shoulder blades. Well, at least imagine it!

○ Don't swing your arms. Move with control because your rear delts are fragile.

○ Lead with your elbows as you lift your arms to isolate your rear delt.

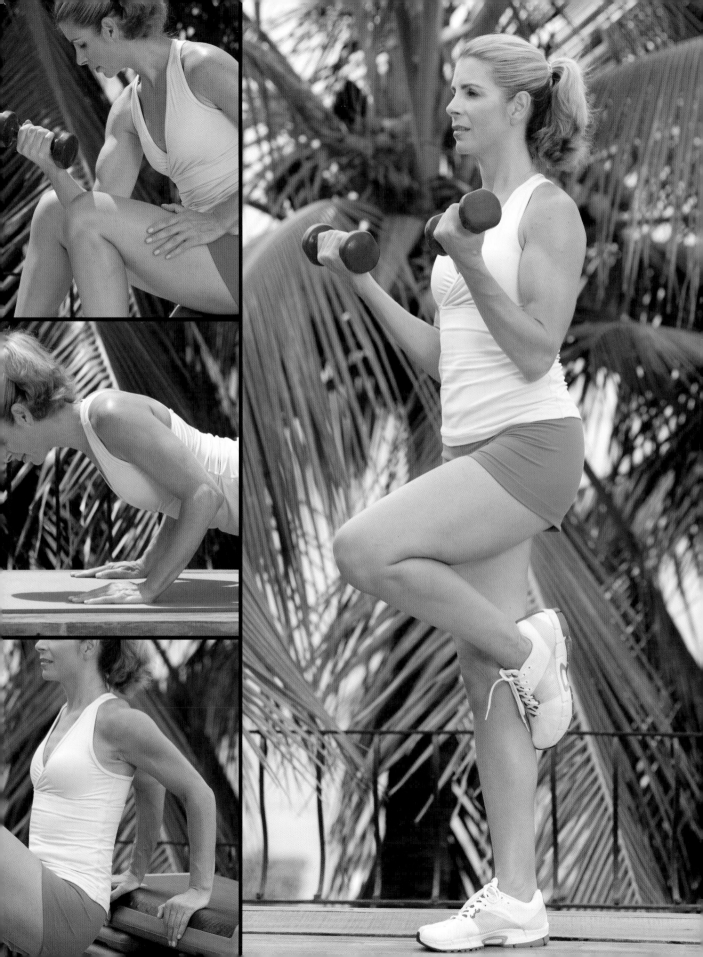

# chapter 11

# AMAZING ARMS

| | | the payoff | total time | how often | sets -n- reps | must-haves |
|---|---|---|---|---|---|---|
| **WORKOUT 1:**<br>beginner<br><br>Triceps Kickback<br>Biceps Curl<br>Triceps Push-Up (Knees) | ○○○○ | Tones the loose skin (urgh—bat wings)! | 15 to 20 minutes | Do this workout 3 times a week on non-consecutive days, such as Mon., Wed., and Fri. | Do three sets of 10 to 12 reps. | Pair of 5- to 10-pound (2- to 4.5-kg) dumbbells |
| **WORKOUT 2:**<br>intermediate<br><br>Overhead Triceps Extension<br>Biceps Concentration Curl<br>Triceps Push-Up | ○○○○ | Let's you say your goodbyes to flabby arms! | 15 to 20 minutes | Do this workout 3 times a week on non-consecutive days, such as Mon., Wed., and Fri. | Do three sets of 12 to 15 reps. | Pair of 5- to 10-pound (2- to 4.5-kg) dumbbells and a step or bench |
| **WORKOUT 3–4:**<br>advanced to super advanced<br><br>Triceps Dip<br>Single-Leg Biceps Curl<br>Single-Leg Triceps Push-Up | ○○○○<br>○○○○ | Leads to superbly toned arms! | 15 to 20 minutes | Do this workout 3 times a week on non-consecutive days, such as Mon., Wed., and Fri. | Do three sets and follow the number of reps given for each exercise. | Pair of 8- to 10-pound (3.5- to 4.5-kg) dumbbells and a step or bench |

# 1 triceps kickback

○○○○

●○○○

**WORKOUT 1:**
# beginner

triceps kickback
biceps curl
triceps push-up (knees)

---

**THE PAYOFF:**
## Tones the loose skin (urgh—bat wings)!

---

**TOTAL TIME:** 15 to 20 minutes

**HOW OFTEN:** Spend two to four weeks building overall strength in your arms. The form is basically the same from exercise to exercise, but do practice! Do this workout three times a week on nonconsecutive days.

★ **AMAZING ARM TIPS,**
on page 203, offers more advice for maximizing this workout.

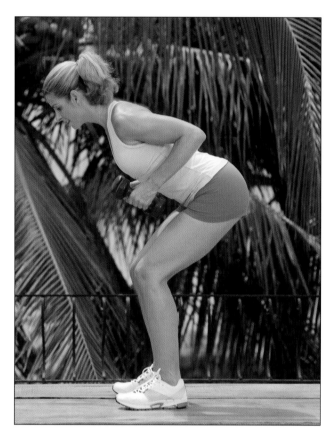

**STARTING POSITION:** Stand in a squat position with a 5- to 10-pound (2- to 4.5-kg) dumbbell in each hand, with your knees bent and hip-width apart. Bend over so that your back is almost parallel with the ground. Bend your elbows to about 90 degrees, raising them to just above your back.

## the payoff:

Gives your arms amazing definition

**sets -n- reps:**  Do three sets of 10 to 12 reps.
**must-haves:**  Pair of 5- to 10-pound (2- to 4.5-kg) dumbbells

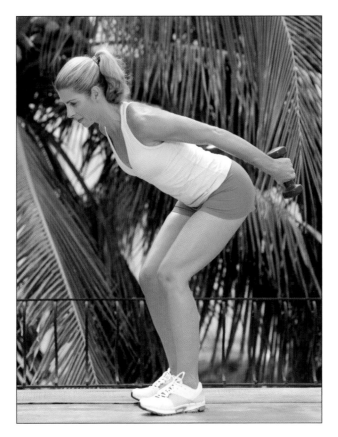

**POSITION 1:** Straighten your arms backward, leading with your little pinky finger. Keep your upper arms stationary and near your ribs. When they're fully extended, your arms should be parallel with the ground. Do 10 to 12 reps.

## FABULOUS FORM TIPS

○  Don't round your spine. Keep your abs active and lengthen your back from the top of your head.

○  Keep your elbows glued to your sides while moving your arms.

○  Fully contract as you straighten your arm, lifting your little pinky a little higher to eke out every ounce of juicy work.

# **1** biceps curl

○○○○

**sets -n- reps:** Do three sets of 10 to 12 reps.
**must-haves:** Pair of 5- to 10-pound (2- to 4.5-kg) dumbbells

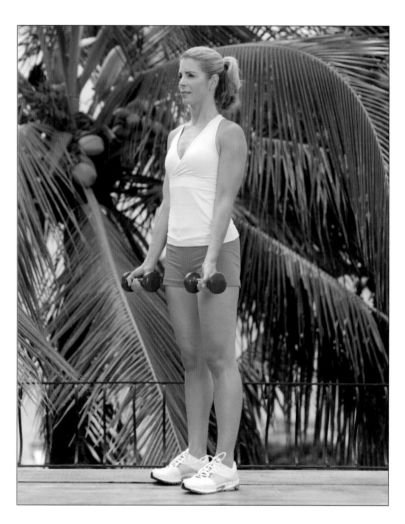

**STARTING POSITION:** Stand with your feet hip-width apart and hold a 5- to 10-pound (2- to 4.5-kg) dumbbell in each hand, palms up. Straighten your arms so the dumbbells rest just outside your thighs.

## the payoff:

Gives you knockout arms!

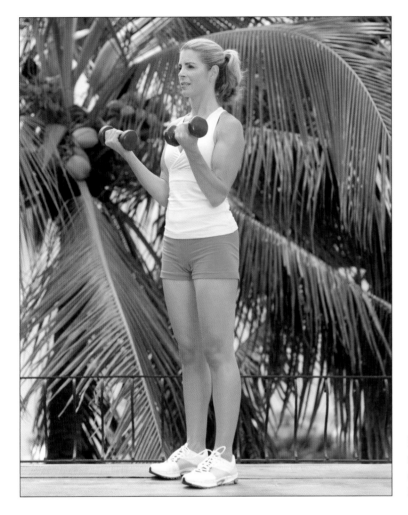

**POSITION 1:** Keep your elbows close to your torso and curl your dumbbells toward your chest. Do 10 to 12 reps.

## FABULOUS FORM TIPS

○ Don't swing your arms as you curl the weight toward your chest.

○ Don't move your elbows; keep 'em glued to your sides to get the full contraction—and lovely arms.

# **1** triceps push-up (knees)

○○○○

| **sets -n- reps:** Do three sets of 10 to 12 reps.
| **must-haves:** Nothing

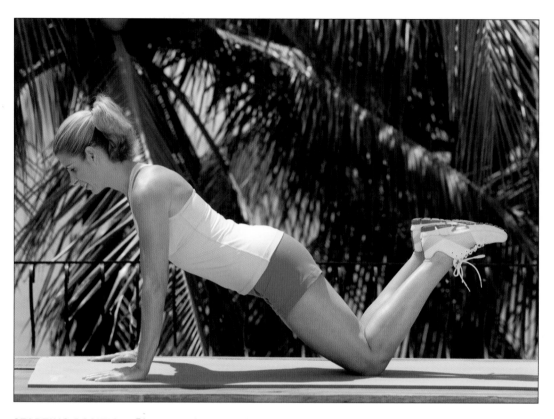

**STARTING POSITION:** Place your knees and hands on the floor so the palms of your hands are directly underneath your shoulders. Lower your body so you're in a plank position.

## the payoff:

Defines your flappage

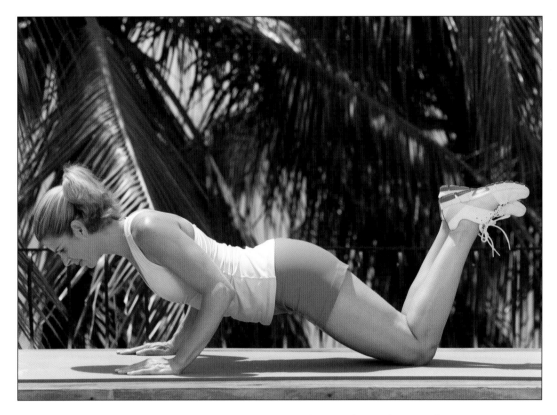

**POSITION 1:** Bend your elbows and point them behind you to lower down until your upper arm and elbow are almost in line with your shoulder. Imagine gluing your elbows to your ribs as you lower and then lift up. Do 10 to 12 reps.

## FABULOUS FORM TIPS

○ Don't splay your elbows out to your sides. They should remain directly by your sides. Imagine a couple of pencils between your arms and ribs. Now squeeze them with your arms.

○ Don't jerk or move too fast. Use controlled movements so as not to put too much pressure on your shoulder girdle.

○ Don't do this exercise if you have a shoulder injury.

○ Don't round your shoulders. To get tips on shoulder placement, turn to page 202.

●●○○○

**WORKOUT 2:**

# intermediate

overhead triceps extension
biceps concentration curl
triceps push-up

**THE PAYOFF:**

## Let's you say your goodbyes to flabby arms!

**TOTAL TIME:** 15 to 20 minutes

**HOW OFTEN:** Spend two to four weeks to beautiful arms. Note: To get rid of the flab, you'll do two different triceps exercises and one biceps exercise. Do this workout three times a week on nonconsecutive days.

★ **AMAZING ARM TIPS,**
on page 203, offers more advice for
maximizing this workout.

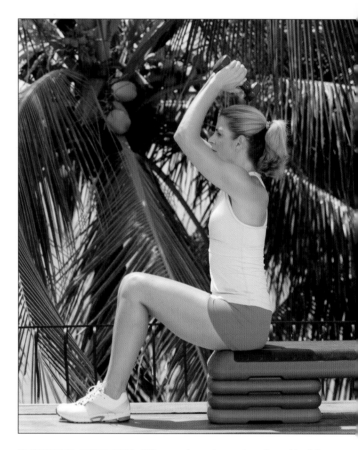

**STARTING POSITION:** Sit on a bench or stand and hold a 5- to 10-pound (2- to 4.5-kg) dumbbell in your hands. Lift your arms over your head and bend your arms so the dumbbell is behind your head, keeping your shoulders down.

## the payoff:

Sculpts the back of your arms

# extension

| | |
|---|---|
| **sets -n- reps:** | Do three sets of 12 to 15 reps. |
| **must-haves:** | Pair of 5- to 10-pound (2- to 4.5-kg) dumbbells and a step or bench |

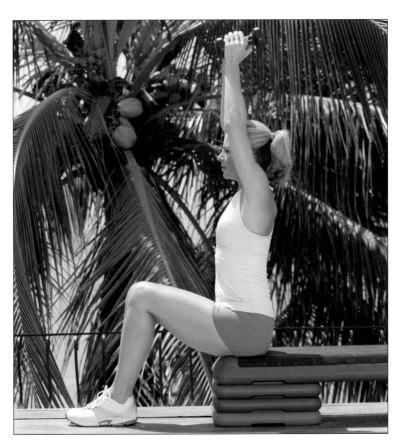

**POSITION 1:** Straighten your arms to the ceiling, leading with your knuckles. Keep your upper arms still so you can fully extend your arms. Do 12 to 15 reps.

## FABULOUS FORM TIPS

○ Don't round your spine. Keep your abs active and lengthen your back from the top of your head.

○ Don't let your shoulders lift toward your ears. Instead, try to relax your upper back.

# **2** biciceps concentration curl

OOOO

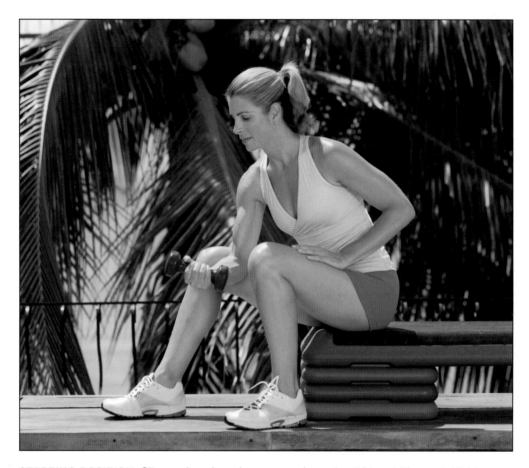

**STARTING POSITION:** Sit on a bench and open your legs about hip-width apart. Hold a 5- to 10-pound (2- to 4.5-kg) dumbbell in your right hand, with your palm up. Bend at the waist and place your right elbow on the inside of your right thigh.

## **the payoff:**

Ultra-sexy arms!

**sets -n- reps:** Do three sets of 12 to 15 reps.

**must-haves:** Pair of 5- to 10-pound (2- to 4.5-kg) dumbbells and a step or bench

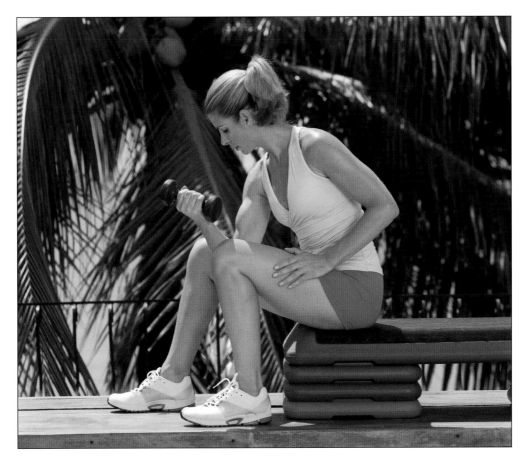

**POSITION 1:** Curl the dumbbell toward your chest. Do 12 to 15 reps, and then switch arms.

## FABULOUS FORM TIPS

❍ Don't swing your arms as you curl the weight toward your chest.

❍ Focus on truly squeezing and contracting your biceps at the top of the movement.

# **2** triceps push-up

**sets -n- reps:** Do three sets of 12 to 15 reps.
**must-haves:** Nothing

○○○○

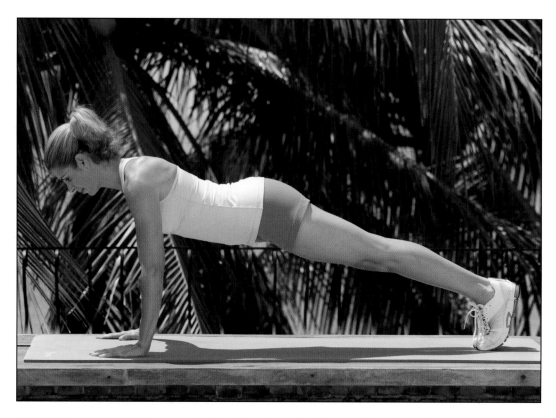

**STARTING POSITION:** Place your feet and hands on the floor so the palms of your hands are directly underneath your shoulders. Lift into a plank position with your belly button to your spine the whole time.

## the payoff:

Eliminates the Bat wings!

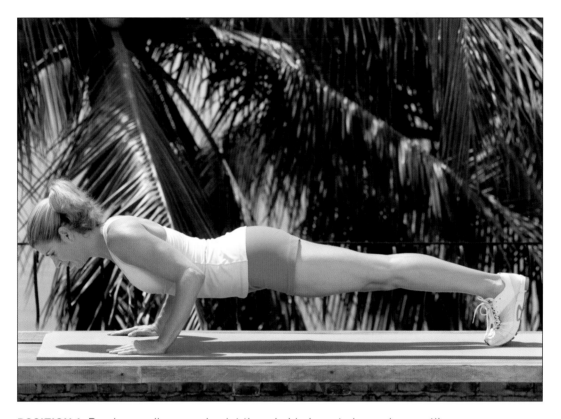

**POSITION 1:** Bend your elbows and point them behind you to lower down until your upper arms and elbows are almost in line with your shoulders. Don't lift your shoulders to your ears. Instead, glue your elbows to your ribs as you lower and then lift up. Do 12 to 15 reps.

## FABULOUS FORM TIPS

○ Don't splay your elbows out to your sides. They should remain directly by your sides. Imagine a couple of pencils between your arms and ribs; now squeeze 'em with your arms.

○ Don't jerk or move too fast. Use controlled movements so as not to put too much pressure on your shoulder girdle.

○ Don't do this exercise if you have a shoulder injury.

○ Don't round your shoulders. To get tips on shoulder placement, turn to page 202.

○ Use your belly to support your lower back. Plus you get a little extra ab work!

○ Only lower down to the point of good form; keep your shoulders down.

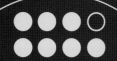

WORKOUT 3-4:

# advanced to super advanced

triceps dip
single-leg biceps curl
single-leg triceps
push-up

---

**THE PAYOFF:**
## Leads to superbly toned arms!

---

**TOTAL TIME:** 15 to 20 minutes

**HOW OFTEN:** Let's up the ante. These exercises challenge your balance, strengthening all the muscles of your ankles, legs, and hips, while "beautifying" your arms. Do this workout three times a week on nonconsecutive days.

★ **AMAZING ARM TIPS,**
on page 203, offers more advice for maximizing this workout.

# 3-4 triceps dip

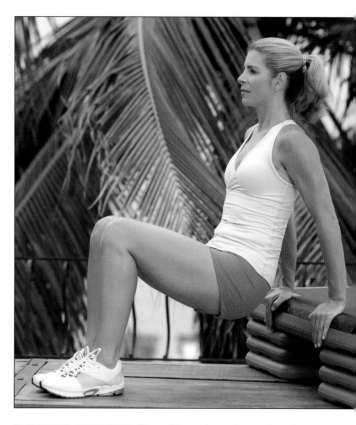

**STARTING POSITION:** Place the palms of your hands on a high bench, and bend your legs in front of your body.

## the payoff:

Arms to die for!

**sets -n- reps:**  Do 15 to 20 reps.
**must-haves:**   A step or bench

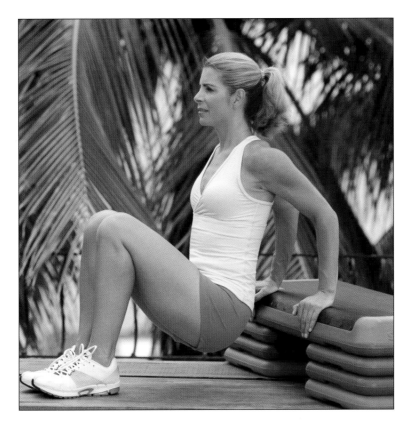

**POSITION 1:** Bend your elbows until your upper arm and elbow make about a 90-degree angle. Imagine that your elbows are kissing as you lower and lift. Do 15 to 20 reps.

## FABULOUS FORM TIPS

- ◯ Don't splay your elbows out to your sides. They should remain directly over your wrists. Imagine them kissing.

- ◯ Don't jerk or move too fast. Use controlled movements so as not to put too much pressure on your shoulder girdle.

- ◯ Don't do this exercise if you have a shoulder injury.

- ◯ Lift your chest.

- ◯ Focus on truly squeezing and contracting your triceps at the top of the movement.

- ◯ If you feel too much pain, pressure, or strain in your shoulders, don't do this exercise. If, on the other hand, this exercise is too easy, straighten your legs.

# 3-4 single-leg biceps curl

○○○○
○○○○

| | |
|---|---|
| **sets -n- reps:** | Do 10 reps. |
| **must-haves:** | Pair of 8- to 10-pound (3.5- to 4.5-kg) dumbbells |

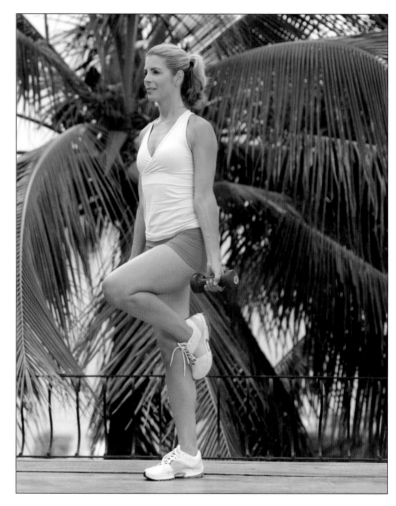

**STARTING POSITION:** Stand with your feet hip-width apart and hold an 8- to 10-pound (3.5- to 4.5-kg) dumbbell in each hand. At the same time, lift your right knee to hip height and lower your arms by your sides. Lengthen from the top of your head to maintain a straight spine.

## the payoff:

Gives you beautiful biceps!

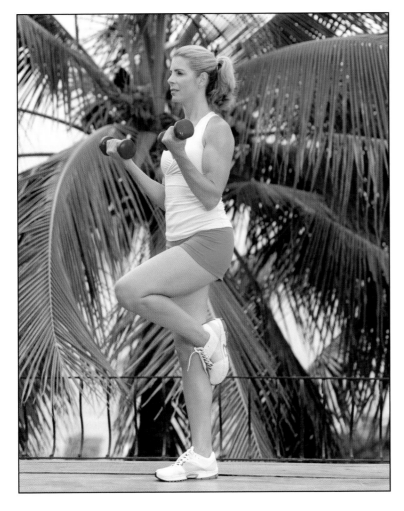

**POSITION 1:** On a count of four, curl your dumbbells to your chest, then slowly lower them. Do 10 reps on each leg.

## FABULOUS FORM TIPS

○ Engage your core muscles to help you balance as you lift the weights.

○ Don't look down. Find a spot on the wall and gaze at it to help you balance.

○ Don't swing your elbows as you curl. Use smooth and controlled movements.

# 3-4 single-leg triceps push-up

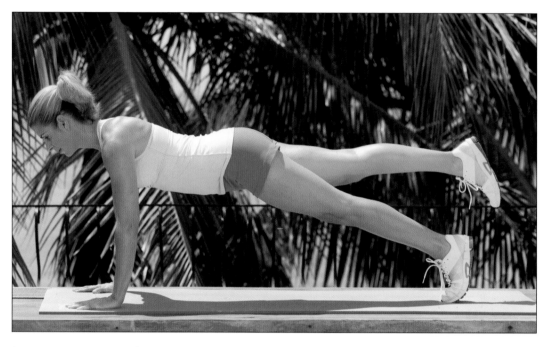

**STARTING POSITION:** Place your feet and hands on the floor so the palms of your hands are directly underneath your shoulders. Lift into a plank position with your belly button to your spine the whole time, and lift your right leg so it lengthens behind you, keeping your hipbones even.

## the payoff:

Blasts the back arm flappage!

**sets -n- reps:** Do three sets of 5-8 reps.
**must-haves:** Nothing

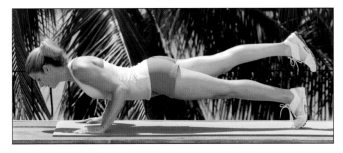

**POSITION 1:** Bend your elbows and point them behind you to lower down until your upper arm and elbow are almost in line with your shoulder. Don't lift your shoulders to your ear. Instead, glue your elbows to your ribs. Do 5 to 8 reps, and then lower your leg to a plank position.

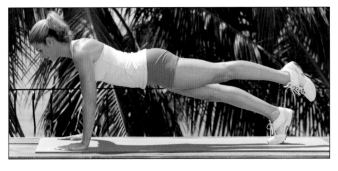

**POSITION 2:** Lift your left leg so it lengthens behind you.

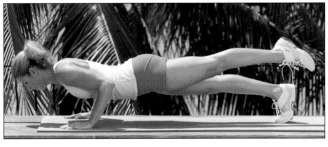

**POSITION 3:** Bend your elbows so they point behind you and lower down until your upper arm and elbow are almost in line with your shoulder. Do 5 to 8 reps.

# FABULOUS FORM TIPS

○ Don't splay your elbows out to your sides. They should remain directly by your sides. Imagine a couple of pencils between your arms and ribs; now squeeze them with your arms.

○ Don't lift your shoulders to your ears; otherwise, you may put too much pressure on your shoulder girdle.

○ Don't jerk or move too fast. Use controlled movements so as not to put too much pressure on your shoulder girdle.

○ Don't do this exercise if you have a shoulder injury.

○ Don't round your shoulders. To get tips on shoulder placement, turn to page 202.

○ Don't lift your leg too high, especially if you want extra booty work.

○ Use your belly to support your lower back—plus you get a little extra ab work!

# List of Exercises

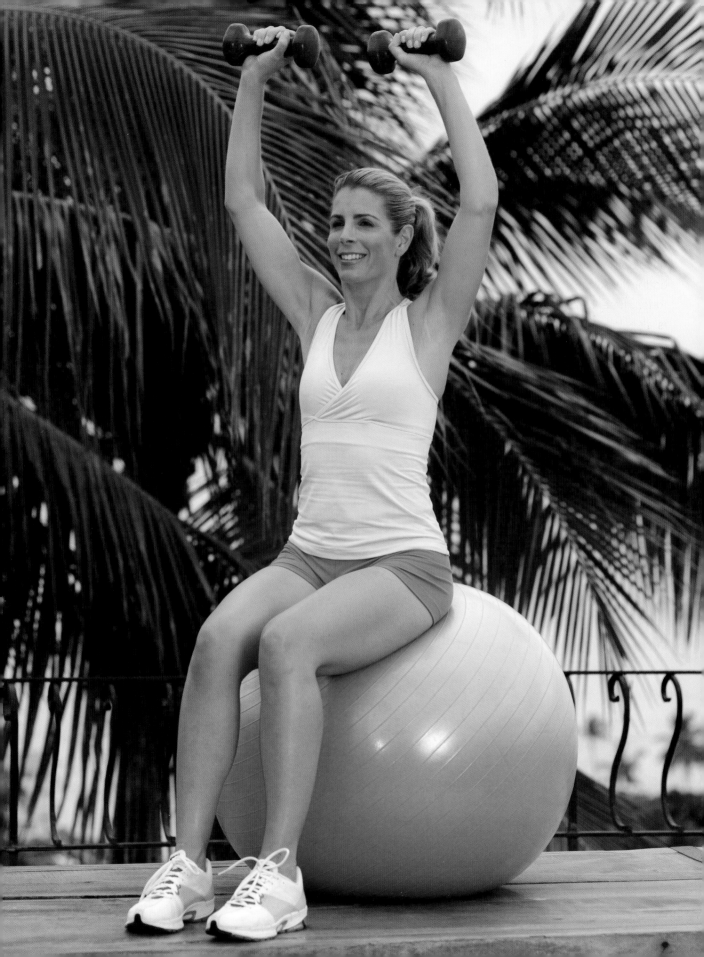

# acknowledgments

**I would like to thank** the usual suspects, such as my awesome and very entertaining publisher, Will Kiester. Of course, the best doesn't stop there! Words can't describe the greatness of the entire Fair Winds editorial team—from my very sweet development editor Cara Connors, to acquisitions editor Jill Alexander, and copy editor Jennifer Bright Reich. I feel like they're my new bbfs—4sure! There is also John Gettings, managing editor, who keeps the wheels turning to make sure my book hits the bookshelves. And then there is Daria Perreault, art director, who is directly responsible for the design of my book. Probably the best in book business is Ken Fund, the "ultraboss," and I'm just so grateful that you keep employing me! Thank you, everybody, for your talent, unparalleled editing, time, well … just everything.

Okay, so I'm totally indebted to Rosalind Wanke, creative director. She is directly responsible for creating some of the prettiest books in the world (yes, seriously). And I'm just honored to work with her along with one of the best photographers in the business, Jack Deutsch. Thank you for being oh-so-sweet and for making me feel gorgeous and helping me look my best (what woman wouldn't want that?). Together, we bonded over the most beautiful scenery and battled tons of mosquitoes in Puerto Vallarta. But … hey, those margaritas made it all so worth it. Thank you, Claudia Rodriquez, for doing my makeup and Fernando Velázquez, Jack's assistant, for going above and beyond and enduring such long workdays. *Muchas gracias*—all!

So, I'm truly a lucky girl. I am blessed to have a wonderful family, friends, students, and an agent who all believe in me and inspire me every day to keep going, even when I just want to check out and find a remote island. (God knows my students would hunt me down.) Thank you for your support, love, and patience.

A special thank you to D.D.!

# about the author

**Karon Karter** is the fitness contributor to Google Docs. She is the author of eight fitness and health books: *The Six-Week Bikini Countdown: Tone Your Butt, Abs, and Thighs Fast Combining Pilates with Select Strength and Cardio Interval Training Workouts*; *Balance Training: Stability Workouts for Core Strength and a Sculpted Body*; *Pilates Lite* (sold in several languages); *The Complete Idiot's Guide to Body Ball Fitness Illustrated*; *The Core Strength Workout*; *The Complete Idiot's Guide to the Pilates Method*; and *The Complete Idiot's Guide to Kickboxing.*

Karon Karter is the host of her own show, *Pilates from the Inside Out*, on Veria, which now airs nationally on the Dish Network. Ms. Karter has been featured in every major newspaper in the country, including the *New York Times*, *Miami Herald*, *Seattle Times*, *Houston Chronicle*, and *Dallas Morning News* (where she is also a special contributor for health and fitness articles). Her books have been publicized in national magazines, including *Shape*, *Self*, *Health*, *Pilates*, the *National Enquirer*, the *Bottom Line*, and *D-Magazine*. She is a frequent health and fitness correspondent to *Good Day Texas* and has made appearances on news shows such as *Good Morning Texas*, *Good Day Phoenix*, and *Fox News*.

She was *Self* magazine's core strength expert for their Self Challenge 2004, where her book, *The Core Strength Workout,* was featured. She was guest author of *Visions: The Women's Expo* (15th Anniversary), where she also put on a Pilates demonstration to hundreds of women. Barnes & Noble featured her books and selected her as the author of the month in January 2005. Ms. Karter has seventeen years' experience in the fitness and health industry, and she interned and then worked for

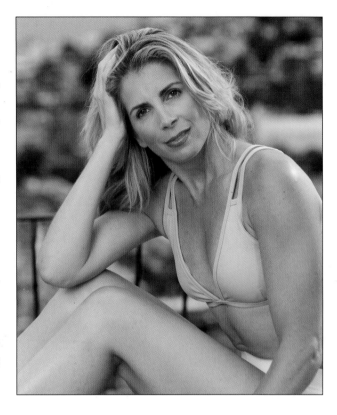

Dr. Kenneth Cooper's Institute for Aerobic Research, where after receiving her BA in corporate fitness she supervised new corporate health programs, such as Dow Chemical's "Up with Life" and Texas Instruments' "Life Track" programs. She has several certifications, including physical fitness specialist and the group leadership from the Aerobics Institute, Resist-a-Ball training, Ashtanga (yoga) training with Manju Jois, Pilates certification from Glenn Studio, and Beryl Bender Birch Ashtanga certification.

Currently, she teaches Pilates and has influenced the fitness lives of thousands of students. You can reach her at www.KaronKarterPilates.com.